Peate's Body Systems

Peate's Body Systems

The Cardiovascular System

Ian Peate, OBE FRCN EN(G) RGN DipN(Lond) RNT BEd(Hons) MA(Lond) LLM

Editor in Chief, British Journal of Nursing;
Consultant Editor, Journal of Paramedic Practice;
Consultant Editor, International Journal for Advancing Practice;
Visiting Professor, Northumbria University;
Visiting Professor, Buckinghamshire New University;
Professorial Fellow, University of Roehampton;
Visiting Senior Clinical Fellow, University of Hertfordshire

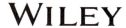

This edition first published 2025.
©2025, John Wiley & Sons Ltd

All rights reserved, including rights for text and data mining and training of artificial intelligence technologies or similar technologies. No part of this publication may be reproduced, stored in a retrieval system, or transmitted, in any form or by any means, electronic, mechanical, photocopying, recording or otherwise, except as permitted by law. Advice on how to obtain permission to reuse material from this title is available at http://www.wiley.com/go/permissions.

The right of Ian Peate to be identified as the author of this work has been asserted in accordance with law.

Registered Office(s)
John Wiley & Sons, Inc., 111 River Street, Hoboken, NJ 07030, USA
John Wiley & Sons Ltd, The Atrium, Southern Gate, Chichester, West Sussex, PO19 8SQ, UK

For details of our global editorial offices, customer services, and more information about Wiley products visit us at www.wiley.com.

Wiley also publishes its books in a variety of electronic formats and by print-on-demand. Some content that appears in standard print versions of this book may not be available in other formats.

Trademarks: Wiley and the Wiley logo are trademarks or registered trademarks of John Wiley & Sons, Inc. and/or its affiliates in the United States and other countries and may not be used without written permission. All other trademarks are the property of their respective owners. John Wiley & Sons, Inc. is not associated with any product or vendor mentioned in this book.

Limit of Liability/Disclaimer of Warranty
The contents of this work are intended to further general scientific research, understanding, and discussion only and are not intended and should not be relied upon as recommending or promoting scientific method, diagnosis, or treatment by physicians for any particular patient. In view of ongoing research, equipment modifications, changes in governmental regulations, and the constant flow of information relating to the use of medicines, equipment, and devices, the reader is urged to review and evaluate the information provided in the package insert or instructions for each medicine, equipment, or device for, among other things, any changes in the instructions or indication of usage and for added warnings and precautions. While the publisher and authors have used their best efforts in preparing this work, they make no representations or warranties with respect to the accuracy or completeness of the contents of this work and specifically disclaim all warranties, including without limitation any implied warranties of merchantability or fitness for a particular purpose. No warranty may be created or extended by sales representatives, written sales materials or promotional statements for this work. This work is sold with the understanding that the publisher is not engaged in rendering professional services. The advice and strategies contained herein may not be suitable for your situation. You should consult with a specialist where appropriate. The fact that an organization, website, or product is referred to in this work as a citation and/or potential source of further information does not mean that the publisher and authors endorse the information or services the organization, website, or product may provide or recommendations it may make. Further, readers should be aware that websites listed in this work may have changed or disappeared between when this work was written and when it is read. Neither the publisher nor authors shall be liable for any loss of profit or any other commercial damages, including but not limited to special, incidental, consequential, or other damages.

Library of Congress Cataloging-in-Publication Data has been applied for.

ISBN: 978-1-394-252350

Cover Images: © marinashevchenko/Adobe Stock, © phototechno/Getty Images, © 4luck/Adobe Stock, © Oleksandr Pokusai/Adobe Stock
Cover Design: Wiley

Set in 9.5pt STIXTwo by Lumina Datamatics

SKY10105420_051225

Contents

Preface viii

Acknowledgements x

1 Anatomy and Physiology: The Cardiovascular System 1

Blood 1
Blood Vessels 6
Heart 10
Conclusion 20
Glossary of Terms 20
Multiple Choice Questions 21
References 23

2 Cardiovascular Assessment 24

The Importance of Cardiovascular Assessment 24
Assessing Needs 25
Chief Complaint and History of Present Condition 27
Family History 27
Lifestyle 28
Past Medical History 28
Physical Examination 28
Palpation 29
The Blood Pressure 33
Chest Examination 34
Electrocardiogram 36
Assessing Chest Pain 39

Conclusion 42
Glossary of Terms 42
Multiple Choice Questions 43
References 44

3 Myocardial Infarction 46

Pathophysiological Changes Associated with Myocardial Infarction 46
Epidemiology 48
Risk Factors 50
Clinical Presentation 51
Clinical Investigations 53
Diagnosis 53
Management 53
Reperfusion 54
Health Teaching 56
Conclusion 57
Glossary of Terms 58
Multiple Choice Questions 59
References 60

4 Heart Failure 62

Pathophysiological Changes Associated with Heart Failure 62
Epidemiology 67
Risk Factors 67
Clinical Presentation 68
Clinical Investigations and Diagnosis 70

Management 72
End of Life Care 73
Health Teaching 73
Conclusion 74
Glossary of Terms 75
Multiple Choice Questions 76
References 77

5 Cardiogenic Shock 79

Cardiac Arrest 79
Epidemiology: Cardiac Arrest 80
Risk Factors Associated with Cardiac Arrest 81
Guidelines for Adult Basic Life Support 81
Shock 83
Shock: Signs and Symptoms 86
Pathophysiological Changes Associated with Cardiogenic Shock 86
Epidemiology 87
Risk Factors 88
Clinical Presentation 89
Clinical Investigations and Diagnosis 89
Potential Investigations 89
Management 90
Health Teaching 90
Conclusion 92
Glossary of Terms 92
Multiple Choice Question 93
References 94

6 Angina 96

Stable Angina 96
Silent Angina 97
Prinzmetal's Angina 98
Microvascular Angina 98

Pathophysiological Changes Associated with Angina 99
Epidemiology 101
Risk Factors 101
Clinical Presentation 103
Clinical Investigations and Diagnosis 103
Management 104
Other Interventions 107
Health Teaching 107
Conclusion 108
Glossary of Terms 109
Multiple Choice Questions 110
References 111

7 Hypertension 113

Primary and Secondary Hypertension 113
Blood Pressure 113
The Cardiac Cycle 115
Pathophysiological Changes Associated with Hypertension 116
Epidemiology 116
Risk Factors 116
Non-modifiable Risk Factors 116
Modifiable Risk Factors 117
Clinical Presentation 118
Blood Pressure Measurement 120
White Coat Syndrome 121
Clinical Investigations and Diagnosis 122
Management 122
Health Teaching 124
Conclusion 124
Glossary of Terms 125
Multiple Choice Questions 126
References 127

8 Peripheral Arterial Disease — 128

Pathophysiological Changes Associated with PAD 128
Epidemiology 130
Risk Factors 130
Clinical Presentation 131
Clinical Investigations and Diagnosis 131
Management 133
Pharmacological Interventions 134
Surgical and Radiological Interventions 135
Amputation 135
Prognosis 136
Health Teaching 136
Conclusion 138
Glossary of Terms 138
Multiple Choice Questions 139
References 140

MCQ Answers — 142

Index — 143

Preface

Welcome to *Peate's Body Systems*; there are 12 books in the series. This is a comprehensive collection of textbooks designed to support and enrich the knowledge of health and care workers across various fields. This series is intended to be a valuable resource for those who are dedicated to understanding the intricacies of human biology, physiology and the various systems that sustain life.

Peate's Body Systems series is rooted in the belief that a deep and thorough understanding of the human body is essential for providing the highest standard of care. Each book in this series is thoroughly crafted to offer clear, accurate and up-to-date information on different body systems. The aim is to bridge the gap between complex scientific concepts and practical, everyday applications in healthcare settings.

PURPOSE AND SCOPE

The purpose of this series is to provide health and care workers with:

- Foundational knowledge, with explanations of the anatomical structures and physiological functions of the body systems

- Insights into how these systems interact with each other and how they are impacted by various diseases and conditions, highlighting clinical relevance and encouraging practical application

STRUCTURE OF THE SERIES

Each book in *Peate's Body Systems* focuses on a specific body system:

The Cardiovascular System	The Female Reproductive System
The Respiratory System	The Male Reproductive System
The Digestive System	The Musculoskeletal System
The Renal System	The Skin
The Nervous System	The Ear, Nose and Throat
The Endocrine System	The Eyes

Every chapter is designed to be comprehensive yet accessible, making complex information easier to digest and apply. Figures, tables, boxes, illustrations and flowcharts have been extensively used to support visual learning and reinforce key concepts.

This series is tailored for:

- Healthcare students: those in nursing and allied health programmes

- Practicing professionals: nurses, therapists and other care workers seeking to deepen their understanding and stay current with the latest developments in health and care

- Educators and trainers: Educators who require reliable and comprehensive teaching materials to advise and instruct the next generation of healthcare providers.

Commitment to Excellence. The series is committed to providing quality educational resources that not only inform but also inspire and empower health and care workers. By equipping you with a robust understanding of the systems of life, you will be better prepared to make informed decisions, deliver compassionate care and ultimately improve patient outcomes.

Thank you for choosing *Peate's Body Systems* as your trusted resource. I hope these textbooks serve as a valuable tool in your ongoing journey of learning and professional development.

IAN PEATE
London

Acknowledgements

I would like to acknowledge the help and support of my partner Jussi Lahtinen. Acknowledgements also go to staff at the RCN Library in London. My thanks go to Tom Marriott, Christabel Daniel Raj, Bhavya Boopathi and all those at Wiley.

Anatomy and Physiology: The Cardiovascular System

CHAPTER 1

The cardiovascular system, also known as the circulatory system, is a complex network of organs and vessels responsible for circulating blood throughout the body. It consists of:

- Blood: the fluid in which materials are transported to and from tissues.
- Blood vessels: the system by which the blood moves to and through tissues and back to the heart.
- Heart: the pump driving blood throughout the body.

Blood provides the fluid environment for the cells of the body with blood vessels transporting the blood. Blood vessels are the network carrying the blood. The heart performs its work as a pump, maintaining blood circulation. The cardiovascular system is essential for maintaining overall health and homeostasis, ensuring all cells receive the necessary oxygen and nutrients whilst removing waste products.

Circulation is key to maintaining organs and tissues. This chapter discusses the anatomy and physiology of the cardiovascular system, the system maintaining blood volume and perfusion of tissues and organs. Understanding how circulation is fundamental to maintaining organs and tissues can help enhance patient care and safety across all spheres of practice.

BLOOD

Through the blood (and lymph) substances are transported around the body; it is the main transportation system of the body, playing a critical role in maintaining homeostasis and supporting the functioning of various body systems. Blood performs three general functions:

1. Transport: transportation of substances around the body, delivering oxygen to every cell.
2. Regulation: blood regulates fluid and electrolyte balance, acid–base balance (pH) and temperature.
3. Protection: clotting factors are present in the blood (thrombocytes), helping protect the body from haemorrhage; blood also contains leucocytes; they help fight infection.

COMPOSITION OF BLOOD

A red sticky fluid, blood is classified as a connective tissue despite its fluid nature. Connective tissues connect, support and bind together various structures and organs in the body. Blood has several different components and can vary slightly from person to person; it can change in response to factors such as hydration, diet and overall health.

Blood consists of formed elements, for example, red blood cells (erythrocytes), white blood cells (leucocytes) and platelets (thrombocytes) (see Table 1.1).

Table 1.1 The three types of blood cells

Blood cell	Description	Role
Erythrocytes	Make up 90% of the formed elements of blood.	Transportation of gases (take oxygen to cells and carry carbon dioxide away from cells).
	Disc shaped (bi-concave).	
	Young red blood cells contain a nucleus (nucleated), while this is absent in mature red blood cells, thereby increasing the oxygen-carrying capacity of the cell.	
	Red in colour due to the presence of the protein haemoglobin (Hb).	
	Formed in the red bone marrow.	
	Life span of approximately 120 days.	
	Old and worn-out erythrocytes are destroyed in the liver and spleen.	
Leucocytes	These are the largest of all blood cells.	Provides the body with protection against infection and disease through the process of phagocytosis (engulfing and ingesting microbes, dead cells and tissues).
	They lack Hb and, as such, are white in colour.	
	Two categories:	
	Granulocytes: Accounting for 75% of white blood cells, further divided into neutrophils, eosinophils and basophils.	
	Agranulocytes: Divided into lymphocytes, 20% of all white blood cells and monocytes account for 5% of white blood cells.	
	Leucocytes often only survive for a few hours but may live for months or years.	
Thrombocytes	Also known as platelets.	Responsible for initiating the blood clotting process leading to the development of blood clots. These blood cells prevent blood loss from a blood vessel by:
	Granular, disc shaped with no nucleus.	
	Small fragments of cells.	
	The smallest cellular elements of blood.	
	Formed in bone marrow.	Gathering where a blood vessel is injured.
	Life span of a thrombocyte is short – five to nine days.	Forming a plug at the injured site and releasing fibrinogen (a chemical) and converting this to fibrin (the net that holds the clot together).

The fluid portion of blood, plasma, contains different types of proteins and other soluble molecules. When a blood sample is separated, the formed elements account for 45% of blood and plasma makes up 55% of the total blood volume. Normally, more than 99% of the formed elements are cells named for their red colour (red blood cells). White blood cells and platelets comprise less than 1% of the formed elements (Figure 1.1). Between the plasma and erythrocytes is the buffy coat, consisting of white blood cells and platelets. See Figure 1.2 for the three formed elements of blood.

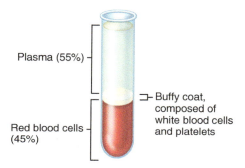

FIGURE 1.1 Appearance of centrifuged blood

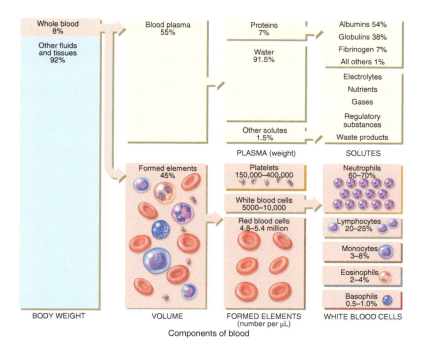

FIGURE 1.2 Three formed elements of blood

The volume of blood is constant unless a person has physiological problems, for example, haemorrhage.

PROPERTIES OF BLOOD

The average adult has a blood volume of approximately 5 L, accounting for 7–9% of the body's weight. Men have 5–6 L and women 4–5 L of blood. Blood is thicker, denser and flows slower than water due to the red blood cells and plasma proteins. Plasma proteins, including albumin, fibrinogen, prothrombin and gamma globulins, make up around 8% of blood plasma in the body (Tortora and Derrickson 2017). These proteins help maintain water balance, affecting osmotic pressure, increasing blood viscosity and helping to maintain blood pressure. The plasma proteins, apart from the gamma globulins, are synthesised in the liver.

Blood has a high viscosity, resisting blood flow. Red blood cells and proteins contribute to the viscosity of blood, which ranges from 3.5 to 5.5 compared with 1.000 for water. Viscosity relates to stickiness of blood; normal viscosity of blood is low, allowing it to flow smoothly. However, the more red blood cells and plasma proteins in blood, the higher the viscosity and the slower the flow of blood. Normal blood varies in viscosity as it flows through the blood vessels; the viscosity decreases as it reaches the capillaries.

Plasma Plasma is a straw-coloured aqueous solution containing plasma proteins, i.e. albumin, globulins and fibrinogen. It also contains inorganic ions regulating cell function, blood pH and osmotic pressure; these include sodium, potassium, chloride, phosphate, magnesium and calcium. Small amounts of nutrients, waste products, drugs, hormones and gases are also found in plasma. Figure 1.3 shows the composition of blood plasma along with the different types of formed elements in the blood.

Plasma is around 91.5% water with 8.5% solutes and most are proteins. Some of the proteins in blood plasma are found elsewhere in the body; those confined to blood are known as plasma proteins. Specific blood cells develop into cells producing gamma globulins, an important type of globulin; these are called antibodies or immunoglobulins, produced during specific immune responses. Other solutes in plasma include electrolytes, nutrients, regulatory substances, such as enzymes and hormones, gases as well as waste products such as urea, uric acid, creatinine, ammonia and bilirubin.

FORMATION OF BLOOD CELLS

Red bone marrow is the primary centre for haemopoiesis. Bone marrow is the soft fatty substance found in bone cavities. Within the bone marrow, all blood cells originate from a single type of unspecialised cell, a stem cell. When a stem cell divides, it first becomes an immature red blood cell, white blood cell or platelet-producing cell. The immature cell divides, matures further and eventually becomes a mature red blood cell, white cell or platelet. Haemopoiesis describes the process by which the formed elements of blood develop (Figure 1.4).

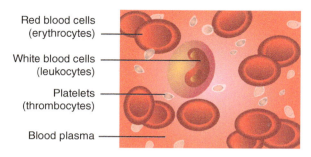

FIGURE 1.3 Components of blood

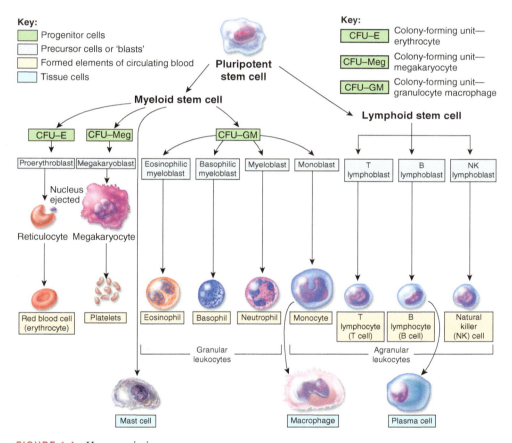

FIGURE 1.4 Haemopoiesis

BLOOD GROUPS

Red blood cells define which blood group an individual belongs to. On the surface of red cells are markers called antigens. Apart from identical twins, each person has different antigens

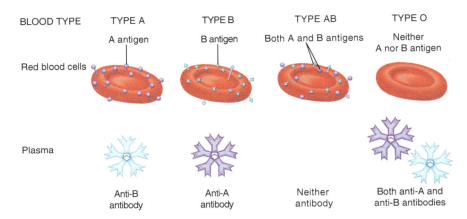

FIGURE 1.5   ABO blood groups

and these antigens are the key to identifying blood types and must be matched in transfusions to avoid serious complications. The structure for defining blood groups is known as the ABO system. If an individual has blood group A, then they have A antigens covering their red cells. Group B has B antigens on their red blood cells, while group O has neither antigens and group AB has both antigens (see Figure 1.5).

The ABO system also covers antibodies in the plasma, the body's natural defence against foreign antigens, for example, blood group A has anti-B in their plasma, B has anti-A and so on. However, group AB has no antibodies and group O has both. If these antibodies find the wrong red blood cells, they attack them and destroy them. Transfusing the wrong blood to a patient can be fatal.

BLOOD VESSELS

Blood vessels are part of the circulatory system transporting blood throughout the body. There are three major types of blood vessels (see Figure 1.6):

1. Arteries carry blood away from the heart.
2. Capillaries enable the actual exchange of water, nutrients and chemicals between blood and tissues.
3. Veins carry blood from capillaries back towards the heart.

The different types of blood vessels are specialised, playing a specific role in circulating the blood around the body.

All arteries, except pulmonary and umbilical arteries, carry oxygenated blood; most veins carry deoxygenated blood from tissues back to the heart; exceptions are the pulmonary and umbilical veins, which carry oxygenated blood. The capillaries form the microcirculatory system; at this point, nutrients, gases, water and electrolytes are exchanged between blood and tissue fluid. Capillaries are tiny, extremely thin-walled vessels acting as a bridge between arteries and veins. The thin walls of capillaries allow oxygen and nutrients to pass from the blood into the tissue fluid and allow waste products to pass from tissue fluid into blood.

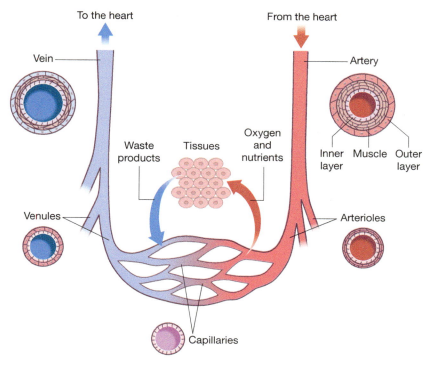

FIGURE 1.6 Blood vessels

STRUCTURE AND FUNCTION OF ARTERIES AND VEINS

In most blood vessels, the walls consist of three layers:

1. Tunica interna (a thin layer of endothelial cells. The epithelial lining is only one cell thick. Therefore, this layer is always very thin.)
2. Tunica media (consists of smooth muscle and elastic fibres).
3. Tunica externa (an outer layer, consisting of fibroblasts, nerves and collagenous tissue).

See Figure 1.7, layers of blood vessels.

ARTERIES

Arteries receive blood under high pressure from the ventricles. They must stretch each time the heart beats, without collapsing under the increased pressure. The walls of arteries have three layers.

1. Outer layer
2. Thick middle layer
3. Inner layer

The outer layer consists of white fibrous connective tissue, merging into the outside with the loose connective tissue. This helps anchor the arteries as the heart pumps the blood

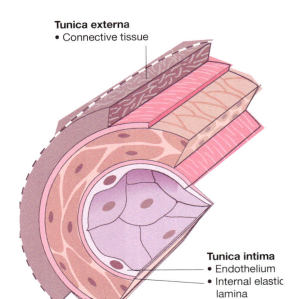

FIGURE 1.7 Layers of blood vessels

through arteries at great pressure (Blanchflower and Peate 2021). The thick middle layer consists of elastic connective tissue and involuntary muscle tissue. This layer is supplied with two sets of nerves: one that stimulates muscles to relax, so the artery is permitted to widen and the other stimulates circular muscles to contract, causing the artery to become narrower. The inner layer of endothelium is made up of flat epithelial cells packed closely together, continuous with the endocardium of the heart. The flat cells make the inside of the arteries smooth to limit friction between blood flowing within the artery and the lining of the vessel.

VEINS

The veins are the major vessels of the venous system. As veins carry blood back to the heart, the pressure exerted by the heartbeat on them is much less than in the arteries. The middle muscular wall of a vein is much thinner than an artery and generally the diameter is larger. Veins also differ from arteries in that they have semilunar valves helping prevent blood from flowing backwards. Figure 1.8 shows a comparison of a vein, artery and capillary.

The vein's valves are necessary to keep blood flowing towards the heart; they are also required to allow blood to flow against the force of gravity; for example, blood returning to the heart from the foot must be able to flow up the leg. Generally, the force of gravity would discourage that from happening. The vein's valves, however, provide 'footholds' for blood as it flows its way up. The valves are like gates, only allowing traffic to move in one direction. They also act with muscle contraction, squeezing the veins and propelling blood towards the heart.

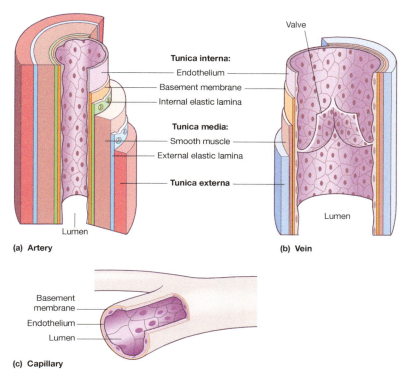

FIGURE 1.8 Comparison of a vein, artery and capillary

Veins receive blood from capillaries after the exchange of oxygen and carbon dioxide has occurred. Veins transport carbon dioxide–rich blood back to the lungs and heart. It is important that carbon dioxide–rich blood keeps moving in the right direction and is not allowed to flow backward; this is accomplished by the semilunar valves present in the veins.

CAPILLARIES

Capillaries are tiny blood vessels of approximately 5–20 μm in diameter. There are networks of capillaries (Figure 1.9) in most organs and tissues. Capillary walls are composed of a single layer of cells, the endothelium. This layer is so thin that molecules such as oxygen, water and lipids can pass through it by diffusion and enter tissues. Waste products such as carbon dioxide and urea can diffuse back into the blood to be carried away for removal from the body. Capillaries are so small, red blood cells must change their shape to pass through them in single file.

The flow of blood in the capillaries is controlled by structures known as precapillary sphincters. These are located between arterioles and capillaries and contain muscle fibres, allowing them to contract. When the sphincters are open, blood flows freely to the capillary beds of body tissue. When the sphincters are closed, blood cannot flow through the capillary beds. Fluid exchange between the capillaries and the body tissues takes place in the capillary bed.

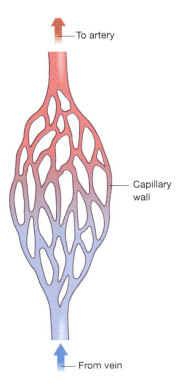

FIGURE 1.9 Capillary network

HEART

This is the hollow muscular pump that forces the movement of blood around the body.

It weighs approximately 250–390 g in men and 200–275 g in women and is about 12 cm long and 9 cm wide. It is in the thoracic cavity (chest) in the mediastinum (between the lungs), behind and to the left of the sternum (breastbone) (Figure 1.10). The heart rests on the diaphragm in the thoracic cavity.

WALLS OF THE HEART

Pericardium A membrane, the pericardium surrounds the heart. This is referred to as a single sac surrounding the heart but is in fact made up of two sacs (fibrous pericardium and serous pericardium) closely connected to each other. These sacs have different structures (Figure 1.11).

Fibrous Pericardium It is a tough, inelastic layer made up of dense, irregular, connective tissue. Its purpose is to prevent overstretching of the heart. It also provides protection to the heart and anchors it in place.

Serous Pericardium It is a thinner, more delicate structure forming a double layer around the heart. The outer layer is fused to the fibrous pericardium. The visceral pericardium (otherwise known as the epicardium) adheres tightly to the surface of the heart.

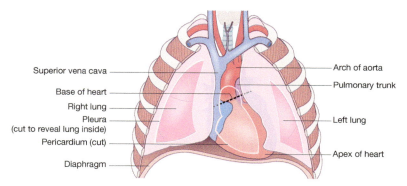

FIGURE 1.10   The location of the heart

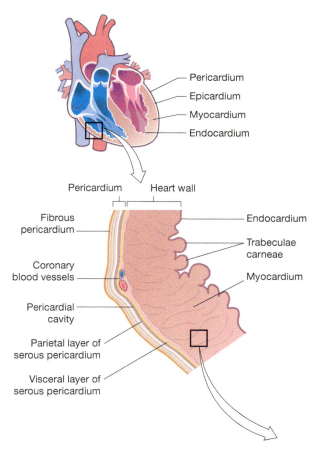

FIGURE 1.11   The walls of the heart

Myocardium   The myocardium makes up most of the bulk of the heart. It is a muscle only found within the heart, specialised in structure and function. The work of the myocardium can be divided into two parts: much of the myocardium is specialised to undertake mechanical work (contraction); the remainder is specialised to undertake the task of initiating and conducting electrical impulses. The cardiac muscle cells (myocytes) are held together in interlacing bundles of fibres arranged in a spiral or in circular bundles (Figure 1.12).

Myocardial thickness varies between all chambers of the heart. Ventricles have thicker walls than atria; however, the left ventricle has the thickest myocardial wall. This is because the left ventricle must pump blood great distances to parts of the body at a higher pressure and the resistance to blood flow is greater.

Endocardium The innermost layer is made up of endothelium overlying a thin layer of connective tissue. The endothelium is continuous with the endothelial lining of the large vessels of the heart. It also provides a lining allowing blood to flow through the chambers smoothly.

CHAMBERS OF THE HEART

The heart has four chambers: two atria (left and right; singular is atrium) and two ventricles (left and right). On the anterior surface of each of the atria is a wrinkled pouch-like structure called an auricle; the main function is to increase the volume of blood in the atrium. Between the ventricles is a dividing wall, the intraventricular septum (Figure 1.13). With the septum between the atria and the septum between the ventricles, there is no mixing of blood between the two sides.

VALVES OF THE HEART

Between the atria and ventricles are two valves (atrioventricular [AV] valves).

- Tricuspid valve – made up of three cusps (leaflets) lying between the right atrium and the right ventricle.
- Bicuspid (mitral) valve – made up of two cusps lying between the left atrium and the left ventricle.

The AV valves prevent the backward flow of blood from the ventricles into the atria.

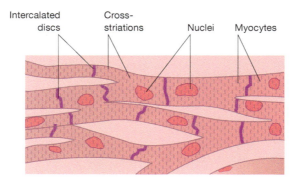

FIGURE 1.12   Cells of the myocardium

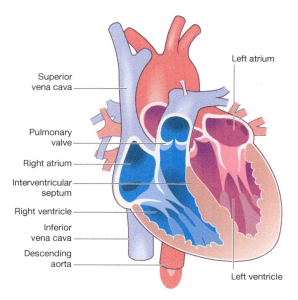

FIGURE 1.13 The chambers of the heart

BLOOD VESSELS OF THE HEART

The aorta is the largest blood vessel of the heart and the largest blood vessel in the body. The aorta carries and distributes oxygen-rich blood to all arteries. The coronary arteries are the first blood vessels branching off from the ascending aorta, supplying richly oxygenated and nutrient-filled blood to the myocardium. There are two main coronary arteries: the right and left coronary artery. Other arteries diverge from these two main arteries, and they extend to the lower portion of the heart.

The pulmonary arteries are unique in that, unlike most arteries transporting oxygenated blood to other parts of the body, pulmonary arteries transport deoxygenated blood to the lungs. After picking up oxygen in the lungs, the oxygen-rich blood is returned to the heart via the pulmonary veins. There are four pulmonary veins extending from the left atrium to the lungs:

1. Right superior vein
2. Right inferior vein
3. Left superior vein
4. Left inferior pulmonary vein

The venae cavae (superior and inferior) (singular vena cava) are the two largest veins in the body, and they carry deoxygenated blood from the various regions of the body to the right atrium. As deoxygenated blood is returned to the heart and continues to flow through the cardiac cycle, it is transported to the lungs where it will become oxygenated. The blood then travels back to the heart and from here it is pumped out to the rest of the body via the aorta. The oxygen-depleted blood is returned to the heart again via the venae cavae.

BLOOD FLOW THROUGH THE HEART

The circulatory system has three distinct parts:

1. Pulmonary circulation (lungs)
2. Coronary circulation (heart)
3. Systemic circulation (systemic)

The heart's parts must work together in a coordinated manner for effective function.

Pulmonary Circulation This is a system of blood vessels forming a closed circuit between the heart and lungs. Blood enters the heart through two large veins, the inferior and superior vena cava, emptying oxygen-poor blood from the body into the right atrium. Blood flows from the right atrium into the right ventricle through the open tricuspid valve. When the ventricles are full, the tricuspid valve shuts. This prevents the blood from flowing backwards into the atria while the ventricles contract (squeeze).

Once the blood travels through the pulmonary valve, it enters the lungs; this is the pulmonary circulation. From the pulmonary valve, blood travels to the pulmonary artery to tiny capillary vessels in the lungs. Here, oxygen travels from the tiny air sacs in the lungs, through the walls of the capillaries, into the blood. At the same time, carbon dioxide, a waste product of metabolism, passes from blood into the air sacs. Carbon dioxide leaves the body as we exhale. Once the blood is oxygenated, it then travels back to the left atrium through the pulmonary veins (Figure 1.14).

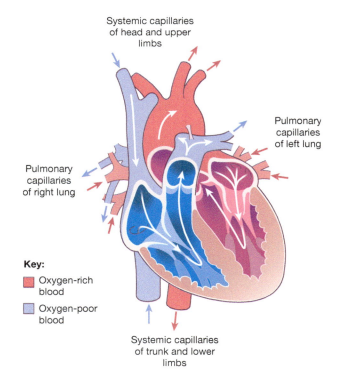

FIGURE 1.14   Blood flow through the heart

Systemic Circulation This is the circuit of vessels supplying oxygenated blood to and returning deoxygenated blood from the tissues. The pulmonary vein empties oxygen-rich blood from the lungs into the left atrium.

Blood leaves the heart through the aortic valve, into the aorta, then to the body (systemic circulation). This pattern is repeated, causing blood to flow continuously to the heart, lungs and body.

The powerful contraction of the left ventricle forces blood into the aorta, which then branches into many smaller arteries running throughout the body. The inside layer of an artery is very smooth, allowing blood to flow quickly. The outside layer of an artery is very strong, enabling blood to flow forcefully. The oxygen-rich blood enters the capillaries where oxygen and nutrients are released. Waste products are collected and the waste-rich blood flows into veins to circulate back to the heart where pulmonary circulation allows the exchange of gases in the lungs to occur.

Coronary Circulation The heart receives about 5% of the body's blood supply. It is essential that the heart receives a plentiful supply of blood to ensure the constant supply of oxygen and nutrients and the efficient removal of waste products required by the myocardium so it performs at an optimum level.

Nutrients from blood cannot diffuse quickly from the heart chambers to supply the cells of the heart. Only the inner part of the endocardium (about 2 mm thick) is supplied with blood directly from the inside of the heart chambers. The rest of the heart's blood supply is supplied by coronary arteries. The coronary arteries come directly off the aorta, just after the aortic valve. They continuously divide into smaller branches and form a web of blood vessels to supply the heart muscle (Figure 1.15).

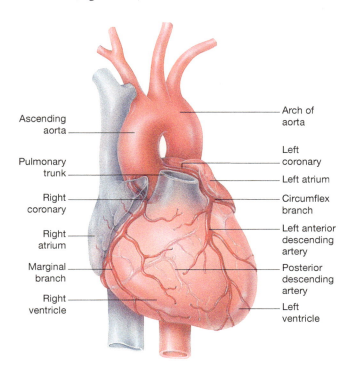

FIGURE 1.15 Blood vessels of the heart

CORONARY ARTERIES

The entire body must be supplied with nutrients and oxygen via the circulatory system; the heart is no exception. The coronary circulation refers to vessels supplying and draining the heart.

Coronary arteries supply blood to the myocardium. As with all other tissues, the heart muscle requires oxygen-rich blood for it to function, and oxygen-depleted blood has to be carried away.

The coronary arteries branch from the ascending aorta, encircling the heart like a crown. As the coronary arteries are compressed during each heart beat, blood does not flow through the coronary arteries at this time. Thus, blood flow to the myocardium occurs during the relaxation phase of the cardiac cycle, the opposite to every other part of the body.

The left coronary artery divides into the anterior interventricular branch, supplying oxygenated blood to both ventricles and the circumflex branch, which distributes oxygenated blood to the left ventricle and left atrium. The right coronary artery divides into the right posterior descending and acute marginal arteries and supplies oxygenated blood to the right atrium and both ventricles, sinoatrial (SA) node (cluster of cells in the right atrial wall regulating the heart's rhythmic rate) and AV node.

CORONARY VEINS

The coronary veins return deoxygenated blood (containing metabolic waste products) from the myocardium to the right atrium. This blood then flows back to the lungs for reoxygenation and removal of carbon dioxide.

Coronary veins contain valves preventing back flow. The coronary sinus is a collection of veins joined together forming a large vessel that collects blood from the myocardium (Figure 1.16). It delivers deoxygenated blood to the right atrium.

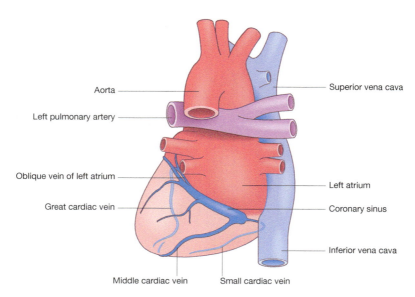

FIGURE 1.16   Coronary veins

The coronary sinus opens into the right atrium, at the coronary sinus orifice, between the inferior vena cava and the right AV orifice. It returns blood from the substance of the heart and is protected by a semi-circular fold of the lining membrane of the auricle.

THE CONDUCTING SYSTEM

The cardiac conduction system is composed of a collection of nodes and specialised conduction cells that initiate and coordinate contraction of the heart muscle. Cardiac conduction is the rate at which the heart conducts electrical impulses. These impulses usually result in the heart contracting and then relaxing. The constant cycle of heart muscle contraction followed by relaxation causes blood to be pumped throughout the body. The conduction pathway is made up of five elements:

1. SA node
2. AV node
3. Bundle of His
4. Left and right bundle branches
5. Purkinje fibres

SA Node The SA node is the natural pacemaker of the heart, located in the right atrium (see Figure 1.17). The SA node is a spindle-shaped structure composed of a fibrous tissue matrix with closely packed specialist cells (Peate 2022). The SA node releases electrical stimuli at a regular rate. The rate at which they are released is determined by the needs of the body. Each stimulus passes through the myocardial cells of the atria, creating a wave of contraction which spreads at speed through both atria.

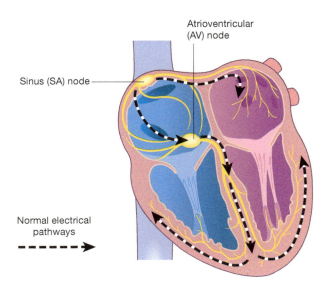

FIGURE 1.17   The conducting system of the heart

The heart is composed of around half a billion cells. The majority of the cells make up the ventricular walls. The rapidity of atrial contraction is such that around 100 million myocardial cells contract in less than one-third of a second, so fast that the contraction of the atria appears instantaneous.

AV Node The AV node is situated on the right side of the partition dividing the atria (see Figure 1.17). When impulses from the SA node reach the AV node, they are delayed for about a tenth of a second. This delay permits the atria to contract and empty their contents first. The AV node regulates the signals to the ventricles, preventing rapid conduction (atrial fibrillation), as well as making sure that the atria are empty and closed before stimulating the ventricles.

Bundle of His Also known as the AV bundle, it is a collection of heart muscle cells specialised for electrical conduction transmitting electrical impulses from the AV node to the point of the apex of the fascicular branches (Nangle 2021). This bundle is the only site where action potentials can be conducted from the atria to the ventricles.

Left and Right Bundle Branches These are the parts of the network of specialised conducting fibres transmitting electrical impulses within the ventricles. Bundle branches are a continuation of the AV bundle, extending from the upper part of the intraventricular septum. The AV bundle divides into a left and a right branch, each going to its respective ventricle by passing down the septum and below the endocardium. Within the ventricles, the bundle branches subdivide, terminating in the Purkinje fibres.

Purkinje Fibres This network of specialised cells is rich with glycogen and has extensive gap junctions; the fibres are located in the inner ventricular walls. They consist of specialised cardiomyocytes that can conduct cardiac action potentials more quickly and efficiently than any other cells in the heart. Purkinje fibres allow the heart's conduction system to create synchronised contractions of its ventricles and are therefore essential for maintaining a consistent heart rhythm.

THE CARDIAC CYCLE

The cardiac cycle is the sequence of events occurring when the heart beats (Figure 1.18). There are two phases of the cardiac cycle. In the diastole phase, the ventricles are relaxed and the heart fills with blood. In the systole phase, the ventricles contract and pump blood to the arteries. One cardiac cycle is completed when the heart fills with blood and the blood is pumped out of the heart.

First Diastole Phase During the diastole phase, the atria and ventricles are relaxed and the AV valves are open. Deoxygenated blood from the superior and inferior venae cavae flows into the right atrium. The open AV valves permit blood to pass through to the ventricles. The SA node contracts, triggering atrial contraction. The right atrium empties its contents into the right ventricle. The tricuspid valve prevents blood from flowing back into the right atrium.

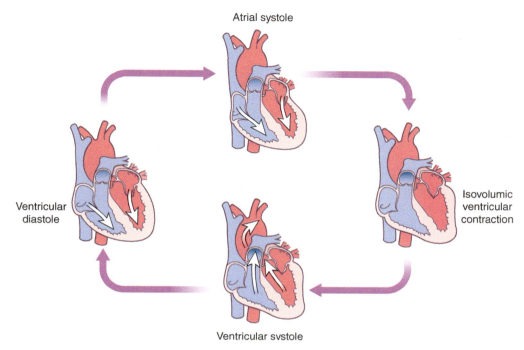

FIGURE 1.18 The cardiac cycle

First Systole Phase During this phase, the right ventricle receives impulses from the Purkinje fibres and it contracts. The AV valves close, and the semilunar valves open. Deoxygenated blood is pumped into the pulmonary artery. The pulmonary valve prevents blood from flowing back into the right ventricle. The pulmonary artery carries blood to the lungs, and gas exchange occurs. Oxygenated blood returns to the left atrium via pulmonary veins.

Second Diastole Phase In the next diastole period, semilunar valves close and AV valves open. Blood from the pulmonary veins fills the left atrium (blood from the venae cavae also fills the right atrium.) The SA node contracts again, triggering atrial contraction. The left atrium empties its contents into the left ventricle. The mitral valve prevents oxygenated blood from flowing back into the left atrium.

Second Systole Phase During the following systole phase, AV valves close and semilunar valves open. The left ventricle receives impulses from the Purkinje fibres and contracts. Oxygenated blood is pumped into the aorta. The aortic valve prevents oxygenated blood from flowing back into the left ventricle. The aorta provides oxygenated blood to all parts of the body. The oxygen-depleted blood is returned to the heart via the venae cavae.

CONCLUSION

The circulatory system is a complex system dealing with the distribution of nutrients, gases, electrolytes, removal of waste products of metabolism and other substances.

This chapter has provided an exploration of the cardiovascular system, seeking to provide readers with a foundation in this sophisticated and vital aspect of human anatomy and physiology.

The cardiovascular system is the lifeline of the body, serving as the transport network for oxygen, nutrients, hormones and waste products. Understanding its structure and function is paramount, as it forms the basis for comprehending a wide range of patient conditions and care interventions. Having insight and understanding of the anatomy and physiology of the cardiovascular system is the cornerstone of your ability to assess patients, interpret diagnostic tests and administer treatments effectively.

This knowledge will be invaluable when assessing heart sounds, detecting irregularities and interpreting electrocardiograms. Haemodynamics and blood pressure are concepts that are critical for comprehending conditions such as hypertension as well as for administering medications and interventions to manage blood pressure effectively. Your understanding will directly impact your practice whether you are monitoring a patient's vital signs, caring for individuals with cardiovascular diseases or assisting in cardiac procedures; this foundational knowledge is indispensable.

Care provision is not just about understanding the science but also about providing compassionate, patient-centred care. Those people with cardiovascular conditions may experience fear, anxiety and vulnerability. Your understanding of the cardiovascular system will enable you to communicate effectively, provide emotional support and deliver holistic care.

In the upcoming chapters, we will further explore cardiac assessments, common cardiovascular disorders, interventions and the art of delivering patient-centred care in the context of cardiovascular health.

GLOSSARY OF TERMS

Aorta: Largest artery in the body, originating from the left ventricle of the heart and carrying oxygenated blood to the systemic circulation.

Arteries: Blood vessels carrying oxygenated blood away from the heart to the body's tissues and organs.

Arterioles: Small branches of arteries that regulate blood flow to the capillaries.

Atria (singular: atrium): Upper chambers of the heart (right atrium and left atrium) that receive blood returning to the heart.

Capillaries: Smallest blood vessels where oxygen and nutrients are exchanged for waste products with tissues.

Cardiac cycle: Sequence of events that occur with each heartbeat, including systole (contraction) and diastole (relaxation) of the heart chambers.

Coronary arteries: Blood vessels that supply oxygen and nutrients to the heart muscle itself.

Diastole: The phase of the cardiac cycle when the heart chambers (ventricles) relax and fill with blood.

Endocardium: Innermost layer of the heart's wall, lining the heart chambers and providing a smooth surface for blood flow.

Endothelium: Inner lining of blood vessels, which plays a role in regulating blood flow and preventing clot formation.

Heart chambers: Atria: Upper chambers of the heart that receives blood.

Ventricles: Lower chambers of the heart responsible for pumping blood to the lungs and the rest of the body.

Heart valves: Atrioventricular (AV) valves: Valves that separate the atria from the ventricles; includes the tricuspid and mitral (bicuspid) valves.

Semilunar valves: Valves located at the exits of the heart; includes the aortic and pulmonary valves.

Myocardium: Middle layer of the heart's wall, consisting of muscle tissue responsible for the heart's pumping action.

Pericardium: Sac-like membrane that surrounds and protects the heart.

Pulmonary artery: Carries deoxygenated blood from the right ventricle of the heart to the lungs for oxygenation.

Pulmonary veins: Carry oxygenated blood from the lungs back to the left atrium of the heart.

Systole: The phase of the cardiac cycle when the heart chambers (ventricles) contract and eject blood.

Veins: Blood vessels that return deoxygenated blood from the body's tissues and organs back to the heart.

Vena cava (superior and inferior): Largest veins in the body, which return deoxygenated blood from the upper and lower parts of the body to the right atrium of the heart.

Ventricles: Lower chambers of the heart responsible for pumping blood; includes the right ventricle and left ventricle.

Ventricular septum: The wall that separates the right and left ventricles of the heart.

Venules: Small veins that collect blood from capillaries and merge to form larger veins.

MULTIPLE CHOICE QUESTIONS

1. Which chamber of the heart pumps oxygenated blood to the systemic circulation?
   a) Left atrium
   b) Right atrium
   c) Left ventricle
   d) Right ventricle

2. What is the main function of the atria in the heart?
   a) Pumping blood to the lungs
   b) Pumping blood to the body
   c) Receiving blood from the body and lungs
   d) Preventing backflow of blood

3. Which blood vessels carry oxygenated blood?
   a) Arteries
   b) Veins
   c) Capillaries
   d) Venules

4. What is the primary function of the coronary arteries?
   a) Carry deoxygenated blood away from the heart
   b) Supply oxygen and nutrients to the heart muscle
   c) Transport blood from the lungs to the heart
   d) Regulate blood pressure

5. During which phase of the cardiac cycle does the heart relax and fill with blood?
   a) Systole
   b) Diastole
   c) Atrioventricular phase
   d) Semilunar phase

6. Which blood vessel carries deoxygenated blood from the right ventricle to the lungs?
   a) Aorta
   b) Pulmonary artery
   c) Pulmonary vein
   d) Superior vena cava

7. What is the term for the phase of the cardiac cycle when the ventricles contract and eject blood?
   a) Systole
   b) Diastole
   c) Atrial depolarization
   d) Ventricular relaxation

8. What is the primary function of capillaries in the circulatory system?
   a) Pump blood to the body's organs
   b) Exchange gases and nutrients with tissues
   c) Prevent backflow of blood
   d) Store excess blood

9. What condition is characterised by the buildup of fatty deposits in the arterial walls?
   a) Atherosclerosis
   b) Hypertension
   c) Angina pectoris
   d) Bradycardia

10. What is the condition characterised by the heart's inability to pump blood effectively?
    a) Bradycardia
    b) Hypertension
    c) Heart failure
    d) Angina pectoris

REFERENCES

Blanchflower, J. and Peate, I. (2021). The vascular system and associated disorders (Chapter 9). In: *Fundamentals of Applied Pathophysiology*, 4e (ed. I. Peate). Oxford: Wiley.

Nangle, V. (2021). The heart and associate disorders (Chapter 8). In: *Fundamentals of Applied Pathophysiology*, 4e (ed. I. Peate). Oxford: Wiley.

Peate, I. (2022). *Anatomy and Physiology for Nursing and Healthcare Students at a Glance*, 2e. Oxford: Wiley.

Tortora, G.J. and Derrickson, B.H. (2017). *Principles of Anatomy and Physiology*, 15e. New Jersey: John Wiley.

CHAPTER 2

Cardiovascular Assessment

This chapter introduces the reader to the key components of assessment related to the cardiovascular system, the techniques involved and the significance of assessment for patient care. Cardiovascular assessment requires a methodological approach to help identify any abnormalities.

Developing essential clinical assessment skills can help provide safe and effective care to patients. One critical aspect of patient assessment is the evaluation of the cardiovascular system. A thorough understanding of cardiovascular assessment is vital as cardiovascular diseases remain a leading cause of morbidity and mortality worldwide.

THE IMPORTANCE OF CARDIOVASCULAR ASSESSMENT

Any dysfunction within this system can have severe consequences for a patient's health and well-being. Therefore, assessing the cardiovascular system is a crucial aspect of patient care, as it aids in the identification of actual and potential issues, monitors disease progression and evaluates the effectiveness of interventions. See Table 2.1 for an overview of where cardiovascular assessment is indicated.

Table 2.1 Areas where cardiovascular assessment is indicated

Sphere of assessment	Implications
Early detection of cardiovascular diseases	Conditions such as hypertension, coronary artery disease, heart failure and arrhythmias often develop silently, progressing slowly. Regular cardiovascular assessments help early identification of risk factors and abnormalities, allowing for timely interventions and preventing complications.
Risk assessment	Cardiovascular assessments are used to evaluate a patient's risk of developing heart-related conditions. By considering factors such as family history, lifestyle choices and physical examination findings, needs are tailored and preventive measures are instigated accordingly.
Treatment planning	Assessment provides crucial information for designing individualised treatment plans. Accurate blood pressure measurements, for example, help determine the choice and dosage of antihypertensive medications, cardiac auscultation findings guide decisions about referrals to cardiologists and the need for further diagnostic tests.
Monitoring chronic conditions	Patients with established cardiovascular diseases require ongoing monitoring to assess the progression of their conditions and the effectiveness of treatment. Regular assessments help make necessary adjustments to medication regimens or lifestyle recommendations.
Pre-operative evaluation	Before surgery, cardiovascular assessments are performed to assess a patient's fitness for the procedure. This can minimise perioperative complications, ensuring a safe surgical experience.

Sphere of assessment	Implications
Emergency situations	In emergency settings, there is a need to quickly assess a patient's cardiovascular status. For instance, in cases of chest pain or arrhythmias, rapid evaluation can be lifesaving. The assessment guides immediate interventions and treatment decisions.
Medication management	Cardiovascular assessments are essential for patients taking cardiac medications. Regular check-ups ensure medications are working effectively and help identify potential adverse effects or drug interactions.
Patient education	Findings from assessments can assist in offering patients information about their condition, risk factors and the importance of adherence to treatment plans. Patient education allows individuals to take an active role in managing their cardiovascular health.
Prevention and health promotion	Assessment is not only about identifying existing issues but also about promoting heart health and preventing future problems. Those who offer care and support can provide guidance on lifestyle modifications, such as diet, exercise, smoking cessation and stress management to reduce cardiovascular risk.
Holistic patient care	Comprehensive healthcare involves looking beyond immediate issues and considering a patient's overall well-being. Cardiovascular assessment is a fundamental part of a holistic approach as it helps to understand how a patient's heart health intersects with their overall health.

ASSESSING NEEDS

A careful and detailed clinical assessment is vital when assessing the probable cause and severity of symptoms, to request appropriate investigations and referrals, to avoid unnecessary investigations and to assess a person's risk of cardiac disease. The way in which the history is taken and information gathered in different healthcare settings varies and depends on, for example, the patient's presenting symptoms, patient concerns and past medical, psychological and social history. The general framework for history taking (see Box 2.1) may need to be amended depending on the care setting (general practice, an acute care setting, a care home or an emergency department) and the nature of the patient encounter (emergency situation or a pre-planned consultation). Many healthcare providers have protocols and procedures for taking a patient history, local policy and procedure must be followed.

BOX 2.1   SYSTEMATIC APPROACH TO HISTORY TAKING

- Presenting complaint
- History of presenting complaint
- Past medical history
- Drug history

(Continued)

BOX 2.1   (CONTINUED)

- Family history
- Social history
- Systems enquiry

Source: Adapted from Bickley (2024); Fairhurst, Innes, and Dover (2023).

The history provides subjective information concerning presenting symptoms, previous patterns of health and illness and the patient's ability to perform the activities of living. A family history, along with risk factor identification and social and psychological background, enriches the history-gathering activity. An in-depth physical examination provides additional objective data.

Explaining to the patient how the history taking will progress, what it entails and how long it may take helps develop rapport and even alleviate anxiety (see Figure 2.1, the usual sequence of events in an examination). Cardiovascular assessment could be considered one of the most important aspects of patient assessment. Throughout the whole assessment process, always be observant of even a slight deviation from the norm. If something is abnormal and uncovered, this warrants further investigation; any findings or concerns must be acted upon and reported.

When meeting the patient, in their own home, a cubicle, in an ambulance, behind screens or in the consultation room, introduce yourself and explain that you will be carrying out an interview and a physical examination. Try to make the patient (and family) relax; the patient may be very anxious, and the provision of a chaperone may be required. Do not rush the patient, give them time as rushing can make them more anxious. Provide time for them to answer questions, do not interrupt when the patient is trying to answer and let them finish before asking the next question.

During the assessment phase, the key is to be as objective as possible; when unsure, further investigation is needed. The use of validated tools along with inspection, palpation, percussion and auscultation provides more credibility for findings and subsequent care delivery. Act on and report findings as clearly as possible. Adhering to local policy and procedure and clearly documenting and communicating findings are essential for the treatment of the patient and the care they receive.

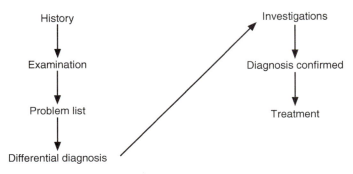

FIGURE 2.1   Usual sequence of events

CHIEF COMPLAINT AND HISTORY OF PRESENT CONDITION

Before performing the assessment, access and read any relevant patient-related data that has already been recorded about the patient, such as notes from any previous admissions. This helps set the screen and contextualise.

The chief complaint and history of the present condition is the story of the illness. Establishing what contributed to the patient coming to the health provider (hospital, general practitioner [GP] practice, walk-in clinic) provides information about the history of the present illness. Seek information regarding present symptoms along with other recent symptoms applicable to this present illness. Obtain the following information specifically associated with the cardiac system:

- Chest and jaw pain
- Pain in the extremities (pain radiating to arms, leg pain or cramps)
- Irregular heart rate or palpitations
- Shortness of breath on exertion when lying down (orthopnoea) or at night (paroxysmal nocturnal dyspnoea)
- Cough
- Cyanosis
- Pallor
- Weakness
- Fatigue
- Unexplained weight changes
- Peripheral oedema
- Dizziness
- Headaches
- Hypo- or hypertension

FAMILY HISTORY

Ask the patient about family history. Ask about the age of any living relatives, including relationships and health of immediate relatives. Ask about hypertension, coronary heart disease, stroke, diabetes, hyperlipidaemia, congenital heart disease and any early deaths in the family before the age of 60 years. A family history can identify those who may have or may be at risk of developing an illness with a genetic component and also provide further information to allow a diagnosis to be made.

The patient's reaction to an illness in the family may influence a response to personal medical problems. A family history of hypertension and myocardial infarction would be included with the history of present illness of a patient with new-onset chest pain. Time limitations may prevent a detailed enquiry into the health of each family member, and use discretion if the family is very large.

LIFESTYLE

Gather details about the current family unit and the nature of the patient's work (to determine physical exertion and stress). How does the patient relax? Do they have any hobbies? Ask about exercise, note type, duration and how often it is undertaken.

Ask about tobacco use and type, age when started and stopped (if at all). How much does the patient smoke? Have there been any attempts to stop smoking? Does the patient drink alcohol, what type, age when they started, how much is consumed (in units) and how often? Is the patient using any recreational (illicit) drugs? How much? How often, which type?

Calculate the patient's body mass index to determine obesity or overweight. Ask about diet.

PAST MEDICAL HISTORY

Exploring past medical history helps to identify any prior diseases or significant factors:

- Ask about hypertension, heart problems, fainting, dizziness or collapses.
- Note if there have been any heart attacks, history of angina and cardiac procedures or operations (type, date of intervention and outcome).
- Previous levels of lipids if checked or known.
- Determine if there is any history of rheumatic fever or heart problems as a child.
- Note any other operations or illnesses, particularly a history of myocardial infarction, hyperlipidaemia, hypertension, stroke or diabetes mellitus.

PHYSICAL EXAMINATION

This is the process of evaluating objective anatomical findings using observation, palpation, percussion and auscultation. Information obtained must be thoughtfully integrated with the history and pathophysiology. This allows an understanding that the aim of the interaction is diagnostic and therapeutic.

Several cardiovascular diseases and disorders have manifestations in systems other than the cardiovascular system and a complete review of other systems should be undertaken whenever possible. The information gained from examining other systems can have a significant impact on decision-making. Perform a general survey, observe the patient as you meet them, noting build (overweight, obesity and wasting), shortness of breath (at rest on exertion), does the patient have difficulty in talking.

Observe the patient. Look at the face and determine: are they pale (pallor), signs of jaundice? Inspect the person's lips and skin: is there any cyanosis? (see Box 2.2.)

BOX 2.2　CYANOSIS

This is a bluish discolouration of the skin caused by a relative decrease in oxygen saturation within capillaries of the skin. Cyanosis in fingers, toes and ear lobes, i.e. peripheral cyanosis, is often related to circulatory problems, such as heart failure. Central cyanosis occurs when more central regions are affected, e.g. tongue, lips and trunk, and it is associated with a lack of oxygenation of arterial blood through the pulmonary system.

Skin colour can reflect overall health, it is an important part of the assessment process, and it may indicate hypoxia. On black or brown skin, it may be easier to see on the palms or the soles. The exact nature of such colour changes, for example, pallor, cyanosis and redness vary with the patient's natural skin colour.

Most skin care guidelines apply primarily to those with light skin, yet care is provided to diverse populations, many from various ethnic backgrounds, with various skin colours.

Source: Adapted from Sommers (2011).

Is there xanthelasma (fatty lumps forming near the inner corners of the upper and lower eyelids, often due to high cholesterol levels)? Is the patient sweaty, do they feel clammy? Table 2.2 outlines common manifestations of cardiovascular problems.

PALPATION

Assess skin temperature, texture and turgor. Check capillary refill, assessing the nail beds on the fingers or toes (see Box 2.3). Capillary refill time should be no more than three seconds. Capillary nail refill test is also known as nail blanch test.

CAPILLARY REFILL TIME

Capillary refill time is a quick and simple test requiring minimal equipment or time to perform and can be measured in any care setting. If there is a prolonged capillary refill time, consider this as a 'red flag', it may identify those at an increased risk of significant morbidity or mortality (see Box 2.3). A slower capillary refill time may indicate a fluid deficit, and a faster

Table 2.2 Common manifestations of cardiovascular problems

System	Manifestation	Potential disorders
General	Fatigue, weight loss, weight gain and disturbed sleep pattern	Coronary heart disease, infective endocarditis, congestive heart failure and valvular disease
Skin	Pyrexia, rigours, skin change in colour/pigmentation, hair loss, oedema, clammy skin and malar flush – redness around the cheeks	Infective endocarditis, pericarditis, peripheral vascular disease, deep vein thrombosis, myocardial infarction and mitral stenosis
Eyes	Visual disturbance (blurred/double), decreased visual acuity, vertigo and headache	Hypertension
Respiratory	Persistent cough (productive, non-productive), pain associated with respiration, dyspnoea, orthopnoea, crackles or wheeze on auscultation	Congestive heart failure, endocarditis and valvular disease
Gastrointestinal	Nausea, vomiting, anorexia, hepatomegaly and splenomegaly	Congestive heart failure, myocardial infarction and congestive heart failure
Musculoskeletal	Arthralgia, jaw pain and back pain	Infective endocarditis myocardial infarction

Source: Adapted from Clare (2022).

one, fluid overload. Delayed capillary refill time according to Dutton and Elliot (2021) is consistent with poor cardiac output.

BOX 2.3   MEASUREMENT OF CAPILLARY NAIL BED REFILL

- Wash hands.
- Explain the procedure; there will be minor pressure on the bed of the nail and this should not cause discomfort.
- Hold the hand to the level of the heart (if using the toe nail bed ensure leg is horizontal).
- Use the finger as the preferred measurement site (toes may also be used).
- Using gentle, but moderate pressure, press for five seconds.
- If possible, measure at room temperature (between 20 °C and 25 °C).
- Allow time for skin temperature to acclimatise if the patient has been moved recently from a warmer or colder environment.
- Count the seconds taken for the nail bed to regain its original colour.
- Normal capillary refill is two seconds or less; an abnormality occurs in three seconds or more.
- Record measurements using the actual number of seconds, for example, capillary refill time is 'four seconds' or 'two seconds or less'.
- If needed, assist the patient to a comfortable position.
- Wash hands.
- Report and document findings.

Remove coloured nail polish before this test. Pressure is applied to the nail bed until it turns white, indicating blood has been forced from the tissue (blanching). Once the tissue has blanched, pressure is removed, while the patient holds their hand at the level of their heart, measure the time it takes for blood to return to the tissue. Return of blood is indicated as the nail turns back to a pink colour.

PULSE

Taking a pulse (palpating a pulse) is a fundamental aspect of assessment. The most common site is at the wrist where the radial artery can be felt pulsating. Table 2.3 lists the sites of peripheral pulses; see also Figures 2.2–2.5.

During each heartbeat, arteries stretch and relax momentarily, this is the pulse and it should have a regular and consistent rhythm. The pulse originates in the aorta spreading as a 'pulse wave' through all arteries. The farther away from the heart the artery is located, the fainter the pulse. When the blood reaches the capillaries, there is no longer a pulse; pulses cannot be felt in those veins returning blood to the heart.

The pulse is a pressure wave in the wall of the artery. If an artery wall is gently palpated at a pulse point, the pulse of pressure in the arterial wall can be felt as blood is squeezed along with each contraction of the heart. The frequency or rate at which the pulse is felt indicates the rate at which the heart is beating.

Table 2.3 Peripheral pulses

Pulse/Artery	Technique	Comments
Radial artery	Radial side of the wrist	Assess rate, rhythm and volume
	Use tips of the index and middle fingers	
Brachial artery	Medial border of humerus at elbow medial to biceps tendon (on the elbow's side)	Assess rate, rhythm and volume
		Can assess character of pulse
	Use index and middle fingers	This is the pulse used when taking blood pressure measurements
Carotid artery	Carotid pulse is located by placing the second and third finger gently on the patient's trachea, locate the Adam's apple (or cricoid cartilage). Move fingers laterally (sideways) approximately 4–5 cm to sternomastoid muscle mass. Pushing medially, locate the carotid artery	Best for pulse character
		To detect carotid stenosis
		Also used during emergency situations such as cardiac arrest
		Never palpate both carotid arteries simultaneously
Femoral artery	With the patient lying flat and undressed (exposing the groin) (ensure dignity) place the finger directly above the pubic ramus and midway between the pubic tubercle and anterior superior iliac spine (between hips and groin)	This is the most easily felt pulse
		To assess cardiac output
		To assess peripheral vascular disease
	Draw an imaginary line from the hip bone to pubic bone, just above the natural crease in the body where the lower abdomen meets the thigh	
Popliteal artery	Located in the knee, back of the leg deep within the popliteal fossa	Used mainly to assess peripheral vascular disease
	Gently palpate against the posterior aspect of distal femur with knee slightly flexed	Popliteal pulse may be difficult to palpate because the artery lies deep in other structures
Dorsalis pedis	Place fingers just lateral (towards the side) to the extensor tendon of the great toe, move fingers more laterally if needed	Used mainly to assess peripheral vascular disease
	With fingers in position linger on the site, varying pressure may assist in picking up a weak pulsation	

Source: Peate (2020). With permission of John Wiley & Sons.

The strength (or amplitude) of the pulse depends on the volume of blood squeezed out of the heart with each beat, known as the stroke volume. The strength of the pulse is influenced by the extent of elasticity of the artery wall.

As a person ages arteries become stiffer (arteriosclerosis), and the extent to which they can stretch with each pulse reduces (Lowry and Ashelford 2015). Cook, Shepherd, and Boore (2021) suggest that the normal value associated with a pulse ranges between 60 and 100 beats per minute (bpm) in a very fit and healthy person, this is 40–60 bpm.

32 CHAPTER 2 Cardiovascular Assessment

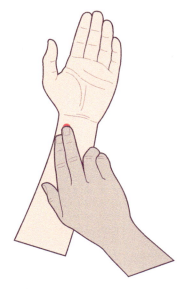

FIGURE 2.2   Assessing the radial pulse

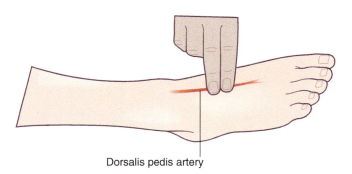

FIGURE 2.3   Palpating the dorsalis pedis pulse

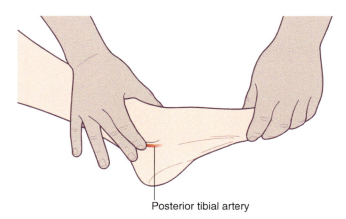

FIGURE 2.4   Palpating the posterior tibial pulse

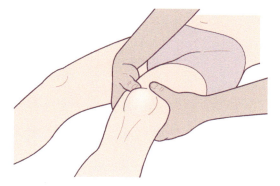

FIGURE 2.5   Palpating the popliteal pulse

Usually, the pulse is easy to palpate; in patients with a weak or unstable pulse, they should be assessed further. A weak pulse can indicate reduced cardiac output and may progress to deterioration. Pulses should be assessed on each side and should be equal and strong.

The rhythm of the pulses should be regular and consistent; an unstable or irregular pulse may suggest irregular contractions of the heart and should be referred to a senior clinician. A patient with a strong, bounding pulse may have high blood pressure. The pulse is assessed for the rate, rhythm and volume and is counted for one full minute. The peripheral pulses can be felt at various sites. See Table 2.3 and Figure 2.6.

Deciding which pulse needs examining depends on individual patient circumstances and whether there are specific clinical reasons for examining a specific pulse or there may be a need to systematically examine all arterial pulses. Usually, the radial pulse is assessed first. However, routinely following this with an examination of the larger brachial and carotid arteries to feel the nature of the arterial wall and particularly the character of the pulse can also be useful.

Increases in pulse rate (tachycardia) could suggest hyperthyroidism, anxiety, infection or anaemia. Slowing of the pulse rate (bradycardia) may be seen in heart block, hypothyroidism or associated with certain drugs (e.g. digoxin, propranolol). Irregularities in the pulse suggest the presence of premature beats and a pulse completely irregular implies the presence of atrial fibrillation. Diminished or absent pulses in various arteries examined could indicate impaired blood flow due to a number of conditions.

A systematic examination of the pulse provides much information, and it is an essential part of clinical practice. Any abnormalities must be reported and acted upon. Results obtained through the measurement of the pulse may lead to further examination of the rest of the cardiovascular system.

THE BLOOD PRESSURE

Blood pressure is a valuable guide to cardiovascular risk, providing essential information concerning haemodynamic status. Blood pressure varies constantly in response to the environment, excitement and stress.

Blood pressure is usually measured in the brachial artery, using a cuff around the upper arm. A large cuff must be used for those who are obese; using a small cuff will result in blood pressure being overestimated. In some instances (the intensive care unit), blood pressure is measured using an invasive device such as an indwelling intra-arterial catheter connected to a pressure sensor.

34 CHAPTER 2 Cardiovascular Assessment

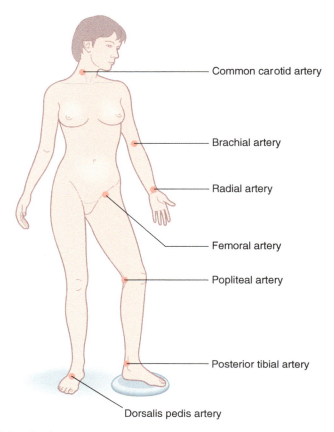

FIGURE 2.6 Peripheral pulses

In patients complaining of chest pain, or if the radial pulses seem asymmetrical, the pressure should be measured in both arms, a difference between the two could indicate aortic dissection (National Institute for Health and Care Excellence [NICE] 2022). Blood pressure is measured in mmHg and recorded as systolic/diastolic.

CHEST EXAMINATION

Several techniques can be used to examine the chest, but not all are discussed here. Identifying the cardiovascular landmarks, understanding and locating these can help detail findings. Explain to the patient what is to be done and why. You may need assistance as you assess the chest. Chest wall inspection can reveal scars that could indicate previous cardiac surgery or pacemaker implantation. Determine if there are any chest wall deformities, for example, funnel chest. Note if the chest moves equally (symmetry); inequality of expansion is often the result of respiratory disease. Take note of the respiratory rate, rhythm and depth. Measure pulse oximetry (NICE 2022).

Ask the patient to breathe out, using both palms of your hands, rest them lightly on the side walls of the chest with thumbs meeting in the middle, then ask the patient to breathe in. Assess the expansion of the chest in full inspiration by noting how far your thumbs move apart. Observe and palpate the trachea, and detect any deviation to the left or right (note any thyroid swelling).

Palpate and percuss to identify any areas of dullness (fluid or lung collapse). Do this by palpating with the flat hand over the fifth intercostal space to feel the maximum impulse (apex of the heart) and note its position; the apex is better defined by the light use of two fingers (noting rib space and its position relative to an imaginary line dropped from the middle of the clavicle).

CARDIAC AUSCULTATION

Auscultation of the heart is an important skill that can take time to master and perform competently. Using the correct technique is essential to distinguish the normal from the abnormal; see Box 2.4 using a stethoscope for auscultation (digital stethoscopes are also available). All cardiac areas must be auscultated and undertaken in a structured and methodical way.

BOX 2.4 USE OF A STETHOSCOPE FOR AUSCULTATION

- A simple stethoscope has a diaphragm or an open bell-shaped structure, applied to the body, connected by rubber or plastic tubes to shaped earpieces for the examiner.
- Prior to using a stethoscope, explain to the patient what you are about to do, and seek consent.
- Use the stethoscope during auscultation to assess breath and heart sounds.
- Hold the diaphragm of the stethoscope firmly against the patient's skin to listen for high-pitched sounds.
- Hold the bell of the stethoscope lightly against the skin to listen for low-pitched sounds.
- Never auscultate over clothing, i.e. a gown, a bra, a vest.
- It may be helpful to close your eyes during the auscultation to help concentrate.
- Note intensity and location of auscultation, document according to local policy.
- Infection prevention and control principles apply when using a stethoscope.

Source: Adapted from Haro and Oliveria (2012).

Cardiac auscultation can identify deviations in blood flow through the valves in the heart. Blood flowing through the heart and the closing of heart valves produces sounds that can be heard when a stethoscope is placed on key areas of the chest wall (see Figure 2.7). The clearest sounds are S1 (first heart sound heard), caused by closure of the mitral and tricuspid valves, heralding the onset of systole and S2 (second heart sound), produced by aortic and pulmonary valves closing, marking the beginning of diastole. Damaged and leaky valves cause a turbulent flow and produce murmurs heard in the quiet time between systole and diastole (Jones, Higginson, and Santos 2010).

The patient should be seated and leaning forward to auscultate heart sounds. If heart signs are faint, ask the patient to lie on their left side, bringing the heart nearer to the chest wall. When auscultating for heart sounds, place the stethoscope over the four sites in Figure 2.7, following the numbered sequence. Auscultation sites are denoted by the names of the heart valves, located along the pathway blood takes as it flows through the heart chambers and valves.

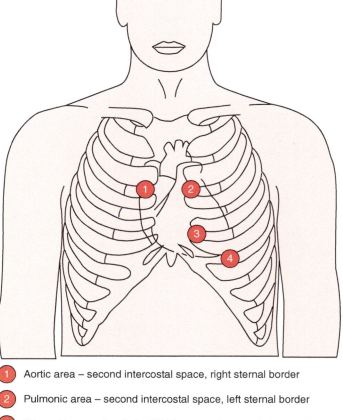

① Aortic area – second intercostal space, right sternal border
② Pulmonic area – second intercostal space, left sternal border
③ Tricuspid area – fourth (or fifth) intercostal space, left sternal border
④ Mitral area or apex – fifth intercostal space, left midclavicular line

FIGURE 2.7 Cardiac auscultation points

Comprehensively assessing cardiovascular status and identifying problems early can put appropriate interventions in place, and, if required, escalate care in a timely manner, helping prevent further deterioration, or arrange for transfer to a more appropriate care area.

ELECTROCARDIOGRAM

Electrocardiogram (ECG) is a recording of the heart's electrical activity. The 12-lead ECG provides a definitive diagnosis measuring electrical activity from a three-dimensional perspective. Information that the 12-lead ECG provides serves as a basis for which other diagnostic tests may be required (for example, echocardiogram).

A 12-lead ECG should be recorded at the earliest opportunity, almost immediately, showing tell-tale signs of cardiac dysfunction, for example, ischaemia and infarction. The 12-lead ECG is an essential criterion for diagnosing acute coronary syndromes. The ECG is a quick and non-invasive approach to acquiring data to determine information about the heart's electrophysiology (Marieb and Hoehn 2023). A two-lead ECG is a basic monitoring technique providing a less detailed view of basic heart rhythm and is used as a continual process (real time). This approach only shows the activity of the heart from one viewpoint at a time. Prior to recording a 12-lead ECG:

- Wash hands/disinfect.
- Explain the procedure.
- Seek consent.
- Check each electrode is attached and correctly placed.
- Ask the patient to lie still and not speak whilst recording.
- Adhere to local policy and procedure.
- Follow guidance issued by NICE (2016).

To record a 12-lead ECG, six electrodes are placed across the front of the chest on the left side. This provides a series of views of the left ventricle as observed from the right side of the heart around to the left side (see Figure 2.8).

Four electrodes are placed on the limbs, placed either on the extremities (ankles and wrists) or on the torso (upper chest and lower abdomen). It is important they are placed symmetrically (see Figure 2.9).

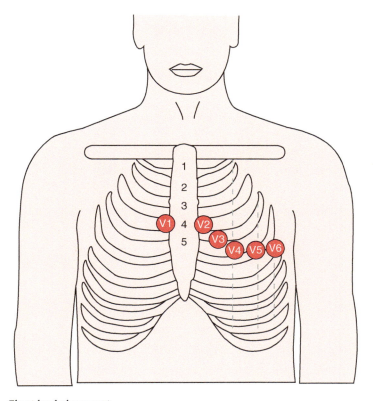

FIGURE 2.8   Chest lead placement

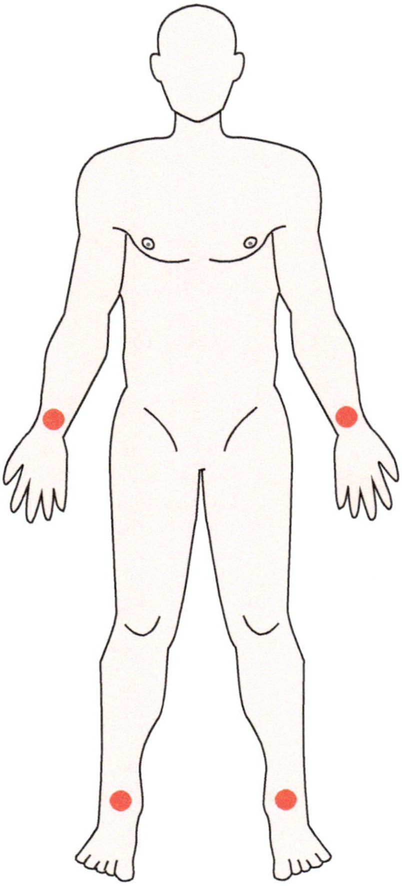

38 CHAPTER 2 Cardiovascular Assessment

FIGURE 2.9 Placement of limb leads

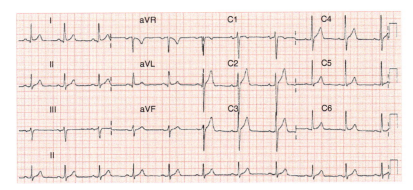

FIGURE 2.10 12-lead normal electrocardiogram. *Source:* Davey (2008). With permission of John Wiley & Sons.

There are 12 views of the heart obtained: six views of the heart from the sides, top and bottom (on the vertical plane); six are views of the anterior surface of the left ventricle (on the horizontal plane). See Figure 2.10 for a normal ECG.

See Box 2.5, when performing an ECG.

BOX 2.5 PERFORMING AN ELECTROCARDIOGRAM (ECG)

- ECG machine should be checked, charged and ready for use.
- There should be sufficient paper for the recording – tissues, clinical wipes, alcohol wipes and a container for disposing of used items.
- Confirm patient identity.
- Female patients should be asked to remove tights and offered a cover for their chest once electrodes and ECG leads are placed and connected.
- Patients with hairy chests may be required to have electrode areas shaved, with permission, ensuring good skin contact.
- The skin should be cleaned and dried, according to local procedure and protocol, before placing electrodes.
- Lie the patient flat, if this is not possible, the back of bed may be raised, this must be noted on the ECG.
- Limb electrodes placed on the limbs – not the trunk.
- Ideally, arm electrodes at the wrist and limb electrodes at the ankles.
- If the person has an amputation or has a dressing in place, electrodes should be placed further up the affected limb but on the same side.
- After the recording, electrodes and leads must be cleaned with clinical wipes according to local procedure and policy.

Source: Houghton and Roebuck (2015); Menzies-Gow (2018).

ASSESSING CHEST PAIN

Cardiac pain is intense and a rapid response is required. Chest pain is a common symptom, one of the most common presenting complaints seen in primary and secondary care; the leading cause of emergency department visits after abdominal pain (Cutungo 2022). A structured assessment can identify those who are at high risk of further complications. The initial aim of the assessment is to identify or exclude a serious cause of chest pain requiring immediate hospital admission, for example, acute coronary syndrome (NICE 2022). Acute coronary syndrome is a potentially more serious cause of chest pain that requires a rapid response in identifying this type of pain and to implement treatment to preserve myocardial function and prevent the development of arrhythmias, heart failure or cardiogenic shock.

It can be challenging to assess and distinguish between various types of chest pain and presentation due to variation in clinical presentation, patient's history of the symptoms, as well as the potential for atypical presentation in women, older people and those with diabetes or chronic kidney disease. Some causes of chest pain are outlined in Table 2.4.

Usually, cardiac chest pain is visceral; it is a deep and diffuse pain as opposed to localised and superficial pain. When asking the patient to locate the pain, typically they point to a wide area of the chest, often being unable to point to a specific point. Cardiac chest pain varies in location depending on each individual. However, it is generally felt in the centre of the chest (or to the left of the sternum) (NICE 2016). It can extend down to the epigastrium or up to the neck and jaw. In some cases, there is a pattern of referred pain extending down the

Table 2.4 Possible causes of chest pain

System	Potential cause
Cardiovascular	Myocardial infarction, unstable angina pectoris, pericarditis, dissecting aortic aneurysm and myocarditis
Pulmonary	Pleurisy, pulmonary embolism, pneumothorax and pneumonia
Haematological	Sickle cell anaemia
Musculoskeletal	Costochondritis and trauma
Gastrointestinal	Gastro-oesophageal reflux, peptic ulcer disease, gallstones and pancreatitis
Non-organic	Anxiety and depression

Source: Adapted from Harskamp et al. (2019); Ball et al. (2023).

Table 2.5 OLDCARTS chest pain assessment

Onset	When did the pain begin?
Location	Where is the pain?
Duration	How long does the pain last?
Characteristics	Describe the pain (crushing, stabbing, dull ache, indigestion).
Associated factors	Other symptoms associated with the pain such as nausea and/or vomiting, weakness, fatigue, breathlessness, syncope (fainting), cold and clammy?
Relieving factors/radiation	Does the pain radiate down the arm or into the neck? Any relieving factors, for example, does it stop when activity stops, is it relieved by sitting forward or resting?
Treatment/temporal factors	Use of vasodilators: i.e. glyceryl trinitrate, is pain relieved by rest or a decrease in physical activity? When does the pain come on? Is pain comparable to previous chest pain?
Severity (intensity)	Use a numerical pain scale (1 no pain – 10 worst pain experienced) to gauge pain severity.

left arm. It should be noted not everybody will experience chest pain in acute coronary syndromes. Those with diabetes mellitus are particularly likely not to experience chest pain due to neuropathy accompanying their condition.

When assessing chest pain, focus on the history of the pain, cardiovascular risk factor profile, a previous personal history of ischaemic heart disease and prior relevant investigations (Cutungo 2022). There are many types of chest pain assessment tools available. Table 2.5 uses the mnemonic OLDCARTS as a framework when assessing chest pain.

In assessing chest pain, effective use of communication is essential, including verbal and non-verbal communication. The person experiencing excruciating chest pain who is fearful for their life may not want to, or not be able to, communicate in depth about their pain. A systematic approach is required when using assessment tools to help make the assessment as objective as possible. Assessment must be augmented by assessing vital signs, ECG and relevant bloods; this aids diagnosis, identifying risk as well as suggesting treatment options.

Chest pain is associated with other clinical pathologies, a thorough assessment of chest pain is required to exclude a non-cardiac cause. Table 2.6 helps interpret what the patient is saying about chest pain and the inferences that can be made regarding causation.

Figure 2.11 provides information related to areas where cardiac pain may be experienced.

Assessing Chest Pain

Table 2.6 Inferences that may be made regarding cardiac pain

The patient says it is:	Possible cause	Location of pain
Aching, squeezing, pressure, heaviness, burning pain, usually subsides within 10 minutes	Angina pectoris	Substernal, may radiate to the neck, jaw, back and arms
Tightness, pressure, burning, aching pain, maybe accompanied by shortness of breath, diaphoresis, weakness, fatigue, anxiety and nausea. 'Feels like a tight belt across my chest'. Sudden onset lasts between 30 minutes and 2 hours. A feeling of impending death	Acute myocardial infarction	Usually across the chest, may radiate to neck, jaw, back and arms
Sharp, continuous sudden onset	Pericarditis	Substernal may radiate to the neck or left arm
Excruciating pain, tearing pain, sudden onset and blood pressure difference in right and left arms	Dissecting aortic aneurysm	Retro sternal, upper abdomen, epigastric may radiate to back, neck and shoulders
Sudden stabbing-like pain, may be accompanied by cyanosis, dyspnoea, cough and haemoptysis	Pulmonary embolism	Over the lung area
Sudden and severe pain can be accompanied by dyspnoea, tachycardia. Breath sounds decreased (particularly over one side)	Pneumothorax	Lateral chest
Burning feeling after eating, may be accompanied by haematemesis, melaena; sudden onset may subside after 20 minutes	Peptic ulcer	Epigastric
Dull stabbing pain, may be accompanied by hyperventilation, breathlessness or sudden onset can last a minute or for several days	Acute anxiety	Anywhere in the chest and neck

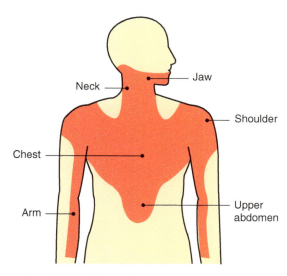

FIGURE 2.11 Areas associated with cardiac pain

CONCLUSION

Experiencing chest pain may result in anxiety for the patient and family. How this is managed can alleviate concerns and anxiety; work in a calm and systemic way. Mastering skills required to undertake an assessment of the person with cardiovascular needs assists in the provision of high-quality care, an ability to detect cardiovascular problems early and contribute to better patient outcomes requires practice. By combining a thorough patient history, physical examination techniques and an understanding of the cardiovascular system's significance, it promotes cardiovascular health and overall well-being.

GLOSSARY OF TERMS

Atrial fibrillation: A type of irregular heart rhythm (arrhythmia) that occurs when the upper chambers of the heart (the atria) beat chaotically and out of sync with the lower chambers (the ventricles). This irregular beating can lead to poor blood flow throughout the body.

Blood pressure: The force exerted by circulating blood on the walls of the blood vessels. It is measured in millimetres of mercury (mmHg) and recorded as two numbers: systolic pressure over diastolic pressure.

Bradycardia: A slower-than-normal heart rate, typically defined as fewer than 60 beats per minute or bpm in adults.

Capillary refill time (CRT): The time taken for colour to return to a capillary bed after pressure is applied and released. It is used to assess peripheral circulation and perfusion.

Diastole: The phase of the cardiac cycle when the heart relaxes and the ventricles fill with blood. Diastolic pressure is the lower number in a blood pressure reading.

Dyspnoea: Difficulty or discomfort in breathing, often associated with heart or lung conditions. It can be a sign of heart failure or other cardiovascular issues.

Heart rate: The number of heartbeats per minute. It can be measured manually by palpation or with an electronic monitor.

Hypertension: High blood pressure, defined as a sustained BP of 140/90 mmHg or higher. It is a major risk factor for cardiovascular diseases.

Hypotension: Low blood pressure, typically defined as a sustained BP below 90/60 mmHg. It may indicate poor perfusion and cardiovascular compromise.

Palpation: The process of examining the body by touch, particularly to assess the size, shape, firmness or location of structures beneath the skin. In cardiovascular assessment, it can involve feeling for pulses or other signs of circulatory function.

Peripheral oedema: Swelling of tissues, usually in the lower limbs, due to fluid accumulation. It can be a sign of heart failure or other cardiovascular issues.

Pulse: The rhythmic expansion of an artery caused by the contraction of the heart. It is often felt at sites where arteries are close to the skin, like the wrist or neck.

Systole: The phase of the cardiac cycle when the heart contracts and pumps blood out of the ventricles. Systolic pressure is the higher number in a blood pressure reading.

Tachycardia: A faster-than-normal heart rate, typically defined as more than 100 bpm in adults.

Vasoconstriction: The narrowing of blood vessels, which increases blood pressure. It can be a response to cold, stress or certain medications.

Vasodilation: The widening of blood vessels, which decreases blood pressure. It can occur in response to heat, relaxation or certain medications.

Venous return: The flow of blood back to the heart through the veins. It is influenced by factors like venous pressure, blood volume and the muscle pump action of the limbs.

MULTIPLE CHOICE QUESTIONS

1. What is the normal range for an adult resting heart rate?
   a) 40–60 bpm
   b) 60–100 bpm
   c) 100–120 bpm
   d) 120–140 bpm

2. Which term describes a heart rate of fewer than 60 bpm?
   a) Tachycardia
   b) Bradycardia
   c) Hypertension
   d) Arrhythmia

3. What does the systolic pressure measure?
   a) Pressure in the veins
   b) Pressure in the arteries during heart relaxation
   c) Pressure in the arteries during heart contraction
   d) Pressure in the lungs

4. What is capillary refill time (CRT) used to assess?
   a) Cardiac output
   b) Peripheral circulation
   c) Heart sounds
   d) Blood pressure

5. Which of the following is a sign of left-sided heart failure?
   a) Peripheral oedema
   b) Jugular venous distension
   c) Dyspnoea on exertion
   d) Ascites

6. Which of the following is NOT a common site to palpate a pulse?
   a) Radial artery
   b) Carotid artery
   c) Popliteal artery
   d) Femoral artery

7. What is the significance of a prolonged capillary refill time?
   a) It indicates normal circulation
   b) It suggests good cardiac output
   c) It may indicate poor peripheral perfusion
   d) It is a sign of hypertension

8. What does a pulse deficit indicate?
   a) The presence of a heart murmur
   b) A difference between the apical and radial pulse rates
   c) A difference between systolic and diastolic pressure
   d) An absence of peripheral pulses

9. What is jugular venous pressure (JVP) used to assess?
   a) Left ventricular function
   b) Right atrial pressure
   c) Peripheral circulation
   d) Cardiac output

10. What does the term 'diastole' refer to in the cardiac cycle?
    a) Contraction of the ventricles
    b) Relaxation of the ventricles
    c) Contraction of the atria
    d) Relaxation of the atria

REFERENCES

Ball, J., Dains, J.E., Flynn, J.A. et al. (2023). Heart (Chapter 15). In: *Seidel's Guide to Physical Examination,* 10e (eds. J. Ball, J.E. Dains, and J.A. Flynn et al.). St Louis: Elsevier.

Bickley, L.S. (2024). *Bate's Guide to Physical Examination and History Taking,* 13e. St Louis: Lippincott.

Clare, C. (2022). The person with a cardiovascular disorder (Chapter 25). In: *Nursing Practice. Knowledge and Care,* 3e (eds. I. Peate and A. Mitchell). Oxford: Wiley.

Cook, N., Shepherd, A., and Boore, J. (2021). *Essentials of Anatomy and Physiology for Nursing Practice,* 2e. London: Sage.

Cutungo, C. (2022). Assessing chest pain. *American Journal of Nursing* 122 (5): 56–58.

Davey, P. (2008). *ECG at a Glance.* Oxford: Wiley.

Dutton, H. and Elliot, S. (2021). The patient with acute cardiovascular problem (Chapter 6). In: *Acute Nursing Care. Recognising and Responding to Medical Emergencies,* 2e (eds. I. Peate and H. Dutton). Harlow: Pearson.

Fairhurst, K., Innes, J.A., and Dover, A.R. (2023). Managing clinical encounters with patients (Chapter 1). In: *Macleod's Clinical Examination,* 15e (eds. A.R. Dover, J.A. Innes and K. Fairhurst). London: Elsevier.

Haro, B. and Oliveria, L. (2012). How to use a stethoscope (Chapter 12). In: *Nursing Profession and Basic Medical Care Techniques World Technologies.*

Harskamp, R.E., Laeven, S.C., and Himmelreich, J.C. (2019). Chest pain in general practice: a systematic review of prediction rules. *BMJ Open* 9 (2): e027081.

Houghton, A.R. and Roebuck, A. (2015). *Pocket ECGSs for Nurses.* London: Taylor & Francis.

Jones, B., Higginson, R., and Santos, A. (2010). Critical care: assessing blood pressure, circulation and intravascular volume. *British Journal of Cardiac Nursing* 19 (3): 153–159.

Lowry, M. and Ashelford, S. (2015). Assessing the pulse rate in adult patients. *Nursing Times* 111 (36/37): 18–20.

Marieb, E.N. and Hoehn, K. (2023). *Human Anatomy and Physiology,* 12e. San Francisco: Pearson.

Menzies-Gow, E. (2018). How to record a 12-lead electrocardiogram. *Nursing Standard* 33 (2): 38–42. doi:10.7748/ns.2018. e11066.

National Institute for Health and Care Excellence. (2016). Recent-onset chest pain of suspected cardiac origin: assessment and diagnosis. https://www.nice.org.uk/guidance/cg95/resources/recentonset-chest-pain-of-suspectedcardiac-ori gin-assessment-and-diagnosis-pdf-975751034821 (accessed September 2023).

National Institute for Health and Care Excellence. (2022). How should I examine a person with chest pain? https://www.nice.org.uk/:~:text=Carry%20out%20a%20physical%20examination%20for%20people%20with,(shock%20and%20arrhythmias).%20Jugular%20venous%20pressure.%20Carotid%20pulse (accessed September 2023).

Peate, I. (2020). *Fundamentals of Assessment and Care Planning for Nurses.* Oxford: Wiley.

Sommers, M.S. (2011). Color awareness: a must for patient assessment. *American Nurse Today* 6 (1): 6.

CHAPTER 3 Myocardial Infarction

Myocardial infarction (MI), commonly known as a heart attack, is a serious medical condition occurring when there is a sudden and prolonged decrease in blood flow to a portion of the heart muscle (myocardium), leading to the death of heart tissue. This can result in various pathophysiological changes.

PATHOPHYSIOLOGICAL CHANGES ASSOCIATED WITH MYOCARDIAL INFARCTION

The pathophysiology of MI and treatment are dynamic and evolving processes and ongoing research continues to deepen understanding of its mechanisms. Early diagnosis, rapid intervention and effective treatments are critical to improving outcomes for individuals experiencing MI; these interventions aim to restore blood flow to the affected area, reduce myocardial damage and prevent complications.

Myocardial infarction is necrosis of a section of myocardial tissue due to ischaemia. Acute MI is historically defined as a clinical syndrome that meets a certain set of criteria, usually a combination of symptoms, electrocardiographic changes and cardiac biomarkers in the proper clinical context. These criteria have evolved and non-invasive and invasive diagnostic imaging and biomarkers have been added (Sandoval, Thygesen, and Jaffe 2020; World Health Organization 2019).

The usual cause of an MI is an atheromatous plaque (caused by coronary heart disease [CHD]) that ruptures or erodes in a coronary artery, causing a thrombus to form (see Figures 3.1 and 3.2). A coronary thrombosis can partially or completely block the blood flow in the artery. Typical features of an MI include severe chest pain, changes on the electrocardiogram

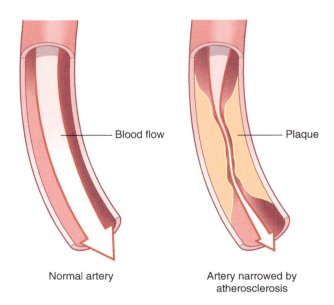

FIGURE 3.1 Atherosclerosis

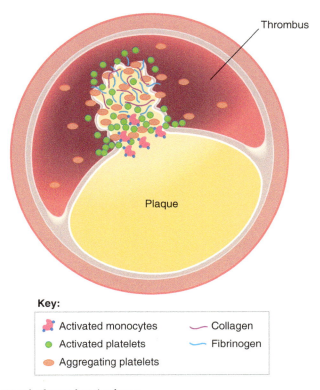

FIGURE 3.2 Ruptured atherosclerotic plaque

(ECG) and raised concentrations of a troponin released from injured cardiac myocytes into the blood. MIs are divided into two types according to the changes they produce on the ECG:

1. ST-segment-elevation MI (STEMI), which is generally caused by complete and persisting blockage of the artery.

2. Non-ST-segment-elevation MI (NSTEMI), reflecting partial or intermittent blockage of the artery.

If a piece of atheroma breaks off, a blood clot forms around this to try and repair the damage to the artery wall. This clot can block the coronary artery (myocardial ischaemia). Myocardial ischaemia results from an occlusion of the coronary artery and oxygen deprivation of the myocardial cells. If the heart muscle is deprived of oxygen for a prolonged period, this may lead to necrosis distal to the occlusion (Figure 3.3). The extent of the ischaemia depends on the location, the extent of the occlusion, the amount of heart tissue supplied by the blood vessel and the duration of the occlusion. It may affect one of the three layers of the heart (pericardium, myocardium and endocardium) or a combination of these layers (Porth 2015).

A collagen scar forms at the position of the infarct and results in the damaged muscle's inability to contract efficiently. Collagen, a bundle of inelastic fibres, does not stretch or contract effectively. Damaged heart tissue conducts electrical signals much more slowly than normal heart tissue; this can result in inefficient contraction of the myocardium, causing:

- A reduction in the volume of blood ejected by the left ventricle with each heartbeat.
- Reduction in cardiac output (volume of blood pumped out by the left ventricle each minute).

48 CHAPTER 3 Myocardial Infarction

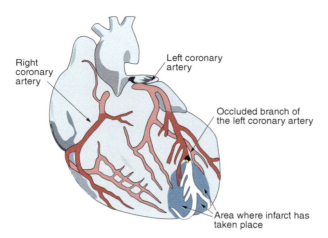

FIGURE 3.3   Myocardial infarction

- Hypotension.
- Reduction in tissue perfusion.

A number of possible complications can occur following an MI, including heart failure, angina, depression and sudden death due to another MI or arrhythmia.

EPIDEMIOLOGY

In the UK, as many as 100 000 hospital admissions each year are due to heart attacks, which is equivalent to 260 admissions each day or one every five minutes. It is estimated that around 1.4 million people living in the UK today have survived a heart attack. This equates to around one million men and 380 000 women (British Heart Foundation [BHF] 2023b). In England, 13.6% of males and 8.3% of females die from ischaemic heart disease (Public Health England [PHE] 2019).

In the UK, the death rates from CHD have fallen by more than half since the early 1960s; then more than 7 of 10 heart attacks were fatal and today, more than 7 out of 10 people survive. This is largely due to primary and secondary preventative strategies as well as percutaneous coronary interventions (PCIs). However, CHD is still one of the leading causes of death in the UK, and, globally, it is the leading cause of death.

YOUNGER PATIENTS

Myocardial infarction often affects patients of older age, and acute MI is gathering more attention as a substantial cause of morbidity and mortality among younger patients, those less than 45 years of age. Krittanawong et al. (2023) note that there is a focus on recognising the unique causes for MI in these younger patients as non-atherosclerotic causes occur more frequently in this age group. As a result, there is a possibility for delayed and inaccurate diagnoses and treatments that may bring with them serious clinical implications. The understanding of acute MI manifestations in young patients is evolving, but there remains a significant need for better strategies to rapidly diagnose, risk stratify and manage such patients.

An important risk factor for MI in young adults is illicit drug use, which is associated with a poor prognosis (Bartolucci et al. 2016). A detailed history of illicit drug use is a necessary part of the assessment of a young person suspected of an acute MI. The most implicated drugs are stimulants that include cocaine, amphetamines and 3,4-methylenedioxy-methamphetamine (MDMA, ecstasy). Cocaine, for example, may increase myocardial oxygen demand because of an increase in blood pressure and heart rate, as well as platelet activation, resulting in acute myocardial ischaemia.

WOMEN

It is a common myth that men and women experience different heart attack symptoms. Indeed, symptoms vary from person to person, but there are no symptoms that women experience more. Mistaken beliefs around symptoms could make women less likely to seek help and receive treatment; this can lead to a delay in diagnosis, resulting in poorer outcomes. Every year in the UK, CHD kills more than twice as many women as breast cancer, despite this, it is often considered a man's disease.

Sex-specific differences exist in the presentation, pathophysiological mechanisms and outcomes in patients with MI. Mehta et al. (2016) noted that cardiovascular disease is an equal-opportunity killer. Sex differences occur in the pathophysiology and clinical presentation of MI and affect treatment delays. Despite more than 30 000 women being admitted to UK hospitals each year with a heart attack, Wu et al. (2018) reported that women had a 50% higher chance than men of receiving the wrong initial diagnosis after an MI. Just like men, there are some women who also fail to recognise the signs and symptoms of a heart attack.

It is important to shift the perception that heart attacks only affect a certain type of person. For example, this is typically an overweight, middle-aged man with diabetes and a smoker. MIs affect the wider spectrum of the population – including women (Wu et al. 2016).

PEOPLE WITH LEARNING DISABILITIES

Data regarding age-related rates of cardiovascular disease in people with learning disabilities is limited and inconclusive. A few studies have analysed the association between learning disability and cardiovascular disease. The prevalence of cardiovascular disease in adults with learning disabilities may be greater and apparent earlier in life than that found in the general population.

People with learning disabilities have increased risks of early-onset cardiovascular disease, particularly for cerebrovascular disease, stroke, heart failure and deep vein thrombosis; risks also increase with the severity of learning disability. These risks have implications for the clinical management of those with learning disabilities and suggest that screening for cardiovascular disease problems could become part of the clinical routine. From a public health perspective, Wang et al. (2023) highlight the importance of cardiovascular disease surveillance and early intervention strategies to enable efficient and effective care among individuals with learning disabilities. The findings discussed by Wang et al. (2023) highlight the importance of an awareness of increased risks of cardiovascular disease in those with learning disabilities.

Risk factors for cardiovascular disease are common in individuals with learning disabilities. Cardiovascular diseases are associated with some genetic causes of learning disabilities. Almost half of all people with Down syndrome, for example, are affected by congenital heart defects.

SOCIAL DEPRIVATION

Cardiovascular disease is a condition that is most strongly associated with health inequalities. Those who live in the most deprived areas are almost four times more likely to die prematurely than someone in the least deprived. There is also a higher prevalence of a number of behavioural risk factors, for example, smoking, physical inactivity, eating fewer than five portions of fruit and vegetables a day and excess weight in more deprived areas compared with less deprived areas (PHE 2018).

ETHNICITY

South Asian and Black groups are at higher risk of cardiovascular disease compared with White groups. Even within these minority groups, there are significant differences in England and Wales, for example, mortality from heart disease is highest among Bangladeshi, Pakistani and Indian groups (Commission on Race and Ethnic Disparities 2021). Globally, South Asians have a higher risk of heart disease. Mortality related to stroke is highest among the Bangladeshi group, and the Black Caribbean, Black African and other Black groups have the highest mortality associated with hypertensive disease. Diabetes prevalence and mortality are highest in all South Asian and Black groups (Raleigh, Jefferies and Wellings 2022).

RISK FACTORS

Cardiovascular health is partly determined by a range of modifiable factors. Around 80% of the cardiovascular disease burden in the UK can be attributed to modifiable risk factors, for example, diet, smoking status and medically manageable risk factors such as hypertension (Dugani et al. 2019). Often, these factors are influenced by a person's ability to access health and care services as well as the social, physical and economic environments in which people live.

The risk factors for cardiovascular disease are also risk factors for other chief causes of morbidity and mortality, for example, diabetes, cancer, dementia and Alzheimer's disease and COVID-19. Cardiovascular disease prevention and management has, therefore, a significant potential for reducing the burden and costs to society of overall morbidity and mortality (Raleigh, Jefferies, and Wellings 2022).

Table 3.1 offers an overview of the key modifiable risk factors for developing cardiovascular disease as well as the non-modifiable factors. Box 3.1 outlines some comorbidities that increase the risk of cardiovascular disease.

Table 3.1 Modifiable and non-modifiable risk factors for developing cardiovascular disease (these are also risk factors for other common conditions, including cancer, diabetes and dementia)

Modifiable	Non-modifiable
Smoking	Age (risk of developing cardiovascular disease increases with age)
Inadequate physical activity	Gender (men have a higher risk of cardiovascular disease than women)
Unhealthy diet	Ethnic background (those from South Asian and Black groups have an increased risk of cardiovascular disease and diabetes)

Modifiable	Non-modifiable
Obesity/overweight	Family history of cardiovascular disease
Excessive alcohol consumption	
	Socio-economic status
	Geographic location

Source: Adapted from Raleigh, Jefferies, and Wellings (2022); BHF (2023).

BOX 3.1 COMORBIDITIES THAT INCREASE THE RISK OF CARDIOVASCULAR DISEASE

- Hypertension
- High or abnormal cholesterol levels or dyslipidaemia
- Irregular heartbeat (atrial fibrillation)
- Hyperglycaemia
- Diabetes
- Chronic kidney disease

Source: Adapted from Raleigh et al. (2022).

CLINICAL PRESENTATION

The clinical manifestations associated with NSTEMI and STEMI are the same. Days to weeks before the event, around two-thirds of patients will have experienced prodromal symptoms, including instability of crescendo angina, shortness of breath and fatigue. Typically, the first symptom of infarction is deep, substernal, visceral pain; this is described as aching or pressure. It often radiates to the back, jaw, left arm, right arm, shoulders or all of these areas (see Figure 3.4). The pain is similar to that experienced in angina pectoris (see Chapter 6 in this book); however, it is usually more severe and long lasting and often accompanied by dyspnoea, diaphoresis, nausea and/or vomiting. It may be relieved temporarily by rest or nitroglycerine. Discomfort may, however, be mild; some acute MIs are silent, meaning they are asymptomatic or may cause vague symptoms that are not seen by the patient as an illness. Some patients will often explain their discomfort as indigestion, particularly because spontaneous relief may be associated with belching or antacid consumption. Some patients present with syncope.

Women are more likely to present with atypical chest discomfort. Older patients may report dyspnoea more than ischaemic-type chest pain.

In severe ischaemic episodes, the patient may have had significant pain, feel restless and worried. Nausea and vomiting can occur. Dyspnoea and weakness as a result of left ventricular failure, pulmonary oedema, shock or arrhythmia may be significant.

The patient's skin can be pale, cool and diaphoretic. There may be peripheral or central cyanosis. The pulse may be thready, blood pressure is variable; however, many patients will initially have some extent of hypertension whilst experiencing pain.

52 CHAPTER 3 Myocardial Infarction

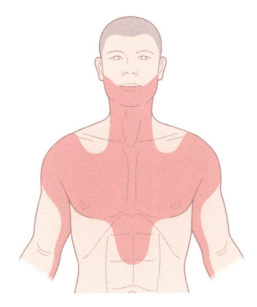

FIGURE 3.4 Areas of pain associated with myocardial infarction

See Box 3.2 for a summary of clinical features.

BOX 3.2   PRESENTATION AND CLINICAL FEATURES

- Chest pain (central chest pain might not be the key symptom).
- Most patients present with characteristic central or epigastric chest pain that radiates to the arms, shoulders, neck or jaw.
- This pain is described as substernal pressure, squeezing, aching, burning or even sharp pain.
- Radiation to the left arm or neck is common.
- The chest pain can be associated with sweating, nausea, vomiting, dyspnoea, fatigue and/or palpitations.
- Shortness of breath: may be the patient's anginal equivalent or a symptom of heart failure.
- Atypical presentations are common; these are usually seen in women, older men, those with diabetes and people from ethnic minorities.
- Atypical symptoms include abdominal discomfort or jaw pain; elderly patients may present with an altered mental state.

Examination can reveal a range of findings and these may vary from person to person:
- Low-grade pyrexia, pale and cool, clammy skin.
- Hypotension or hypertension, depending on the extent of the MI.
- Dyskinetic cardiac impulses (in anterior wall MI) can be palpated occasionally.

- Third and fourth heart sounds, systolic murmur if there is mitral regurgitation or ventricular septal defect develops, pericardial rub.
- There may be signs of congestive heart failure, including:
  - Pulmonary rales
  - Peripheral oedema
  - Elevated jugular venous pressure

CLINICAL INVESTIGATIONS

Depending on the setting, if a diagnosis is suspected and the person is in a community setting, immediately arrange urgent hospital assessment and admission. Where possible, patient history and clinical examination include palpation, auscultation and percussion.

A 12-lead ECG is the most important test and it should be done as soon as possible, within 10 minutes of presentation. Taken together, serial dynamic ECGs may demonstrate progression that is seen during acute MI.

Serial cardiac markers (serum markers of myocardial cell injury) are cardiac enzymes released into the bloodstream after myocardial cell necrosis. These markers appear at different times after injury, levels decrease at different rates.

Full blood count to rule out anaemia. Measure C-reactive protein and other markers of inflammation, renal function and electrolytes, glucose, lipids and clotting screen.

Pulse oximetry and blood gases. Monitor oxygen saturation.

Chest X-ray to assess the heart size and presence or absence of heart failure and pulmonary oedema (can assist in making a differential diagnosis). Other imaging modalities will depend on clinical need (i.e. myocardial perfusion scintigraphy, stress echocardiography). CT coronary angiography if clinical assessment indicates this. Echocardiography helps define the extent of the infarction and assess overall ventricular function, and can identify complications, such as acute mitral regurgitation, left ventricular rupture or pericardial effusion.

DIAGNOSIS

Adults with suspected acute coronary syndrome are assessed for acute MI using the criteria in the universal definition of MI (National Institute for Health and Care Excellence [NICE] 2020; Sandoval, Thygesen, and Jaffe 2020). Diagnosis is by ECG and the presence or absence of serological markers.

MANAGEMENT

If not already done, an intravenous (IV) cannula is inserted. Treatment is antiplatelet drugs, anticoagulants, nitrates, beta-blockers, statins and reperfusion therapy. For STEMI, emergency reperfusion is via fibrinolytic drugs, PCI or, occasionally, coronary artery bypass graft surgery (CABG). For NSTEMI, reperfusion is via percutaneous intervention or CABG surgery.

The initial management of acute MI is based on maintaining patient safety, the reduction of myocardial work and the reperfusion of the heart muscle. The patient is also attached to continuous cardiac monitoring as the risk of cardiac arrhythmias and even cardiac arrest are high. Continuous close clinical monitoring, including symptoms, pulse, blood pressure, heart

54 CHAPTER 3 Myocardial Infarction

Table 3.2 Medication and myocardial infarction (MI)

Medication	Discussion
Antiplatelet agent	Long-term low-dose aspirin reduces overall mortality, non-fatal re-infarction, non-fatal stroke and vascular death.
	Clopidogrel, used with low-dose aspirin, is recommended for acute MI with ST-segment elevation, for four weeks.
	Clopidogrel alone is an alternative when aspirin is contra-indicated.
Beta-blockers	When commenced within hours of infarction, beta-blockers reduce mortality, non-fatal cardiac arrest and non-fatal re-infarction.
	Unless contra-indicated, the usual regimen is to administer intravenously on admission and then continue orally – titrate upwards to the maximum tolerated dose.
Angiotensin-converting enzyme (ACE) inhibitors	ACE inhibitors reduce mortality whether or not patients have clinical heart failure or left ventricular dysfunction. They also reduce the risk of non-fatal heart failure.
	Measure renal function, electrolytes and blood pressure prior to commencing an ACE inhibitor repeat within one to two weeks.
Cholesterol-lowering agents	Ideally, initiate therapy with a statin as soon as possible for all patients with evidence of cardiovascular disease unless contra-indicated.

Source: Adapted from Joint Formulary Committee (2023); BHF (2023a).

rhythm and oxygen saturation by pulse oximetry, oxygen therapy and pain relief, usually in a cardiac care unit. Confident and competent care interventions can help to relieve any anxiety that the patient (and family) may be experiencing.

Chest pain can be treated with nitrates (nitroglycerine) or, depending on assessment, morphine. Nitrates are preferable to morphine, which should be used judiciously, for example, if a patient has a contraindication to nitrates or is in pain despite nitroglycerine therapy. Nitrates are initially administered sublingually, followed by continuous IV infusion if required. Morphine 2–4 mg IV, repeated every 15 minutes as needed, is highly effective; this can, however, depress respiration, can reduce myocardial contractility and is a potent venous vasodilator causing hypotension and bradycardia. It is important to ensure that local policies and procedures are adhered to.

Patients are usually treated and discharged home with the following:

- Angiotensin-converting enzyme (ACE) inhibitors
- Antiplatelet treatments
- Beta-blockers
- Cholesterol-lowering agents (statins)

See Table 3.2, pharmacological agents and MI.

REPERFUSION

Reperfusion refers to the restoration of blood flow to the heart. The patency of the occluded artery can be restored by PCI or by giving a thrombolytic drug. PCI is the preferred method. Compared to a conservative strategy, an invasive strategy (PCI or CABG surgery) is associated with reduced rates of refractory (chronic) angina and rehospitalisation in the shorter term and MI in the longer term (Fanning et al. 2016). There are, however, procedure-related risks associated with reperfusion.

In primary PCI, the patient has a catheter inserted through an opening made in the femoral or radial artery and the catheter is manoeuvred to the coronary artery, where the blockage is located. A balloon is then passed through and inflated, pushing the thrombus into the walls of the artery, if necessary, a metal cage (a stent) is inserted into the artery to keep the artery patent (Clare 2022) (Figure 3.5).

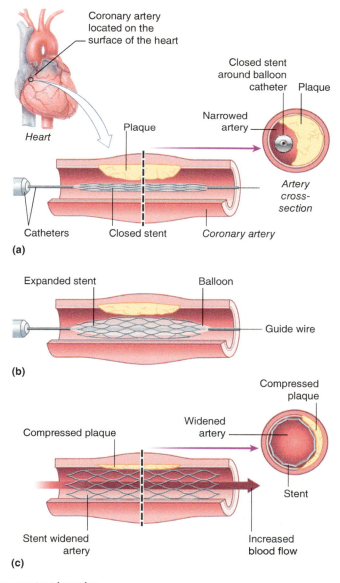

FIGURE 3.5 Coronary stent insertion

HEALTH TEACHING

A patient-centred approach is essential when offering health promotion and this should be documented in the care record. It can take a while to come to terms with having had an MI. Everyone is different; for some recovery will be quick, for others, it can take longer.

Decisions should be made by the patient and full explanations provided with due note taken of the patient's needs and preferences.

Early risk assessment can aid the identification of high-risk patients who may require further management with angiography and coronary revascularisation. Methods of cardiac assessment vary according to local availability and expertise. Several specific risk assessment tools are available.

All people who have had an MI should be given advice about, and offered, a cardiac rehabilitation programme that includes an exercise component. This should commence as soon as possible and should normally be started in the hospital prior to discharge. Healthcare professionals should be aware of what is involved and encourage ongoing participation. Cardiac rehabilitation is an essential part of treatment. The programme is usually run by a team including experienced cardiac nurses, physiotherapists and exercise specialists. The aim is to help the patient recover well and as quickly, as possible. Each programme is different – patients are individually assessed soon after they leave the hospital and commence the programme when it is safe and appropriate, usually this is after about four weeks.

Some concerns that people may have, which may need to be discussed, following an MI are provided in Table 3.3.

Table 3.3 Lifestyle discussion points following an myocardial infarction (MI)

Concern	Information
Returning to work and normal activities	Most people will return to work even though they have been diagnosed with MI. British Heart Foundation (BHF) have produced information: https://www.bhf.org.uk/informationsupport/support/practical-support/work-and-a-heart-condition
Driving	Many people who have a heart condition can continue to drive depending on what sort of heart condition the person has, whether the person is symptomatic and the type of treatment they have had. The Driver and Vehicle Licensing Agency (DVLA) has produced information about health conditions and driving: www.gov.uk/health-conditions-and-driving
Sexual activity	Sex is no more likely to trigger a heart attack than any other form of activity. People resume having sex when they feel ready, usually, this is two to four weeks after a heart attack. If the patient has had surgery, it may be longer.
	Even if the patient does not feel ready for intercourse, other activities such as foreplay and oral sex do not place additional strain on the heart.
Erectile dysfunction	The inability to achieve or maintain an erection may be a side effect of medication. It should also be noted that women can experience a loss of sexual desire. Talking to the practice nurse or general practitioner (GP) about issues experienced could lead to a change or reduction in the dose of medication.

Concern	Information
Air travel	Most people with a heart or circulatory condition can travel safely without risking their health.
	The BHF provides some hints and tips when planning a holiday: https://www.bhf.org.uk/informationsupport/support/practical-support/holidays-and-travel
Stress and anxiety	People may feel stressed, anxious, afraid or uncertain about what is to come.
	Feeling sad, fatigued and worried can be expected after a heart attack; however, these feelings should disperse as the person gets back into a routine. If it does not, encourage the patient to talk to the nurse or GP. Depression is intricately linked to heart disease and can put recovery at risk.
Competitive sport	Recovery from a heart attack is different for everyone. Patients are advised to check with the cardiac rehabilitation team or doctor before returning to or taking up exercise.
	It is important that the patient does not rush or have unrealistic expectations of themselves whilst recovering. Rushing, overdoing it, could delay recovery and newly built confidence could be lost.

Offer the following information to the person who is post MI based on individual assessment:

- Eat a healthy, low-salt diet.
- Adhere to the medication regimen.
- Maintain a healthy body weight.
- Become physically active, register on a cardiac rehabilitation programme.
- Maintain blood pressure, blood glucose and lipids.
- Reduce/do not smoke.
- Attend outpatient follow-up.
- Do not ignore chest pain – call a general practitioner/clinic/emergency services.

CONCLUSION

Understanding MI can equip you with the knowledge necessary to recognise the signs and symptoms, monitor ECG changes and provide effective care for patients experiencing this critical cardiovascular event. Early recognition and intervention can make a substantial difference in patient outcomes. Moreover, remaining aware of the latest research in this field ensures you can deliver the best possible care to patients with cardiovascular diseases, contributing to improved patient outcomes and quality of life.

Myocardial infarction is a serious cardiac event that demands immediate recognition and action. As a student healthcare worker, a thorough grasp of the risk factors, clinical presentation, diagnostic processes and management strategies are essential for providing effective care to correct. Furthermore, educating patients about risk reduction and lifestyle modifications empowers them to take charge of their heart health, contributing to improved outcomes and quality of life.

GLOSSARY OF TERMS

Acute coronary syndrome: A spectrum of conditions, including heart attack, that stop or reduce blood from flowing to heart muscle.

Angina pectoris: Chest pain or discomfort caused by reduced blood flow to the heart muscle, often a precursor to MI.

Arrhythmia: An irregular heart rhythm, which can occur during and after an MI.

Atherosclerosis: A build-up of fatty deposits inside the arteries. The disease is often described as a hardening or narrowing of the arteries.

Cardiogenic shock: A severe condition where the heart is unable to pump enough blood to meet the body's needs, often seen in severe MI cases.

Cardiovascular disease: A collective term for all diseases affecting the heart and blood vessels.

Coronary heart disease: An umbrella term for diseases occurring when the walls of the coronary arteries become narrow caused by a gradual build-up of atheroma. Two main forms of CHD are MI and angina. Also known as ischaemic heart disease (IHD).

Embolus: A clot or other foreign material that travels through the bloodstream and can block a blood vessel, leading to an MI.

Heart failure: A chronic condition occurs when the heart cannot pump blood efficiently around the body. It occurs because the heart has been damaged or is overworked. Some may have few or no symptoms. Those with symptoms experience a range of problems, including shortness of breath, general tiredness and oedema of the feet and ankles.

Ischaemia: A condition where there is an inadequate blood supply to a specific area of the body, such as the heart muscle, which leads to oxygen deprivation.

Infarct: An area of tissue that has died due to a lack of blood supply, as seen in MI.

Myocardial infarction (MI): Also known as a heart attack, occurs when there is a sudden blockage of blood flow to a part of the heart muscle, leading to tissue damage or death.

NSTEMI: Non-ST-segment-elevation MI, a type of MI characterised by less pronounced ECG changes, often indicating partial blockage of a coronary artery.

Percutaneous coronary intervention (PCI): A minimally invasive procedure, such as angioplasty with stent placement, used to open blocked coronary arteries.

Reperfusion: Restoration of blood flow to the heart muscle through treatments like angioplasty and thrombolytic therapy.

Thrombus: A blood clot forming within a blood vessel or the heart.

Troponin: A cardiac enzyme released into the bloodstream when there is heart muscle damage, often used to diagnose MI.

STEMI: ST-segment-elevation MI, a type of MI characterised by significant ST-segment elevation on the ECG, indicating acute and complete blockage of a coronary artery.

Vasodilators: Medications that relax blood vessels, reducing the heart's workload and increasing blood flow, often used in MI management.

MULTIPLE CHOICE QUESTIONS

1. What is another term for MI?
   a) Heartburn
   b) Heart attack
   c) Heart murmur
   d) Heart failure

2. Which of the following is the most common cause of MI?
   a) High cholesterol
   b) Hypertension
   c) Smoking
   d) Diabetes

3. What is the primary cause of MI?
   a) Atherosclerosis
   b) Viral infection
   c) Genetic predisposition
   d) Lack of exercise

4. Which of the following symptoms is NOT typically associated with MI?
   a) Chest pain or discomfort
   b) Shortness of breath
   c) Nausea and vomiting
   d) Muscle cramps

5. What cardiac enzyme is typically elevated in the blood following an MI?
   a) Troponin
   b) Creatinine
   c) Haemoglobin
   d) Platelets

6. Which diagnostic test is often used to confirm the diagnosis of MI?
   a) Electrocardiogram (ECG)
   b) Chest X-ray
   c) Magnetic resonance imaging (MRI)
   d) Blood glucose test

7. What term is used to describe the death of heart muscle tissue due to lack of blood supply?
   a) Cardiomyopathy
   b) Myocarditis
   c) Ischaemia
   d) Infarction

8. What is the most common location for pain or discomfort during an MI?
   a) Left upper arm
   b) Right leg
   c) Left chest or arm
   d) Lower abdomen

9. Which of the following lifestyle factors is NOT a modifiable risk factor for MI?
   a) Smoking
   b) Diet
   c) Age
   d) Physical activity

10. What is the primary goal of reperfusion therapy in the treatment of MI?
    a) To reduce blood pressure
    b) To prevent clot formation
    c) To restore blood flow to the blocked coronary artery
    d) To relieve anxiety

REFERENCES

Bartolucci, J., Nazzal, N.C., Verdugo, F.J. et al. (2016). Characteristics, management, and outcomes of illicit drug consumers with acute myocardial infarction. *Revista Medica de Chile* 144: 39–46.

British Heart Foundation (2023a) Medicines for heart conditions. https://www.bhf.org.uk/information support/treatments/medication (accessed September 2023).

British Heart Foundation (2023b). UK factsheet. https://www.bhf.org.uk/-/media/files/for-profess ionals/research/heart-statistics/bhf-cvd-statistics-uk-factsheet.pdf (accessed September 2023).

Clare, C. (2022). The person with a cardiovascular disorder (Chapter 25). In: *Nursing Practice. Knowledge and Care*, 3e (eds. I. Peate and A. Mitchell). Oxford: Wiley.

Commission on Race and Ethnic Disparities. (2021). Ethnic disparities in the major causes of mortality and their risk factors – a rapid review. https://www.gov.uk/government/publications/the-report-of-the-commission-on-race-and-ethnic-dispar ities-supporting-research/ethnic-disparities-in-the-major-causes-of-mortality-and-their-risk-factors-by-dr-raghib-ali-et-al (accessed September 2024).

Dugani, S.B., Ayala Melendez, A.P., Reka, R. et al. (2019). Risk factors associated with premature myocardial infarction: a systematic review protocol. *BMJ Open* 19 (2): e023647. doi:10.1136/bmjopen-2018-023647.

Fanning, J.P., Nyong, J., Scott, I. et al. (2016). Routine invasive strategies versus selective invasive strategies for unstable angina and non-ST elevation myocardial infarction in the stent era. *Cochrane Database Systematic Review* 26 (5): CD004815. doi:10.1002/14651858.CD004815.pub4.

Joint Formulary Committee (2023). British National Formulary (online). BMJ and Pharmaceutical Press. https://bnf.nice.org.uk (accessed September 2023).

Krittanawong, C., Khawaja, M., Tamis-Holland, J.E. et al. (2023). Acute myocardial infarction: etiologies and mimickers in young patients. *Journal of the American Heart Association* 12 (18): e029971. https://doi.org/10.1161/JAHA.123.029971.

Mehta, L.S., Beckie, T.M., and DeVon, H.A. (2016). Acute myocardial infarction in women: a scientific statement from the American Heart Association. *Circulation* 133: 916–947. https://doi.org/10.1161/CIR.0000000000000351.

National Institute for Health and Care Excellence (2020). Acute coronary syndromes in adults. https://www.nice.org.uk/guidance/qs68/esources/acute-coronary-syndromes-in-adults-pdf-2098794360517 (accessed September 2023).

Porth, C.M. (2015). *Essentials of Pathophysiology: Concepts of Altered Health States*, 4e. Philadelphia: Wolters Kluwer.

Public Health England (2018). Health profile for England: 2018 chapter 5: inequalities in health. https://www.gov.uk/government/publications/health-profile-for-england-2018/chapter-5-inequa lities-in-health (accessed September 2023).

Public Health England (2019). Health matters: preventing cardiovascular disease. https://www.gov.uk/government/publications/health-matters-preventing-cardiovascular-disease/health-matters-preventing-cardiovascular-disease (accessed September 2023).

Raleigh, V., Jefferies, D., and Wellings, D. (2022). Cardiovascular disease in England. Supporting leaders to take action. https://www.kingsfund.org.uk/insight-and-analysis/reports/cardiovascular-disease-england (accessed September 2023).

Sandoval, Y., Thygesen, K., and Jaffe, A.S. (2020). The universal definition of myocardial infarction. *Circulation* 141 (18): 1434–1436. doi.org/10.1161/CIRCULATIONAHA.120.045708.

Wang, H., Lee, P.M.Y., Zhang, J. et al. (2023). Association of intellectual disability with overall and type-specific cardiovascular diseases: a population-based cohort study in Denmark. *BMC Medicine* 21 (41): 41. doi.org/10.1186/s12916-023-02747-4.

World Health Organization (2019). International Classification of Diseases. BA41 acute myocardial infarction. ICD-11 for mortality and morbidity statistics. https://icd.who.int/browse11/l-m/en#/http://id.who.int/icd/entity/1334938734 (accessed September 2023).

Wu, J., Gale, C.P., Hall, M. et al. (2016). Editor's choice – impact of initial hospital diagnosis on mortality for acute myocardial infarction: a national cohort study. *European Heart Journal: Acute Cardiovascular Care* 7 (2): 139–148.

CHAPTER 4 Heart Failure

Heart failure is a complex medical condition characterised by the heart's inability to pump blood at sufficient pressure, leading to insufficient oxygen and nutrient delivery to the body's organs and tissues. This condition can result from various underlying causes; it is a syndrome of ventricular dysfunction. Left ventricular failure results in shortness of breath and fatigue, and right ventricular failure causes peripheral and abdominal fluid accumulation. Both ventricles can be involved or separately.

The European Society of Cardiology (2021) notes that heart failure is not a single pathological diagnosis, but a clinical syndrome consisting of cardinal symptoms and signs. It is the result of structural and/or functional abnormalities of the heart resulting in increased intracardiac pressures and/or inadequate cardiac output at rest and/or during exercise.

Clare (2020) explains that heart failure can be acute or chronic and right-sided, left-sided or bilateral. Heart failure is also known as:

- Congestive cardiac failure: right-sided heart failure
- Congestive heart failure: right-sided heart failure
- Left ventricular failure: left-sided heart failure

PATHOPHYSIOLOGICAL CHANGES ASSOCIATED WITH HEART FAILURE

Heart failure is an umbrella term used to describe the inability of the heart to sustain a normal cardiac output that ultimately leads to poor perfusion of tissues. The pathophysiology of heart failure is complex and is the subject of much research. Heart failure can be roughly categorised into three categories.

1. Heart failure due to left ventricular systolic dysfunction: The part of the heart that pumps blood around the body (left ventricle) becomes weak, most commonly caused by CHD, especially myocardial infarction (MI). The incidence of heart failure with reduced ejection fraction (HFrEF) in the UK has reduced as the treatment of MI has improved.
2. Heart failure with preserved ejection fraction (HFpEF): The incidence of HFpEF is increasing in the UK, probably as a consequence of better treatment of MI but also as an effect of an ageing population.
3. Heart failure due to valve disease.

There are a range of intricate pathophysiological changes occurring as a result of heart failure; at the core of heart failure is impaired cardiac function (see Table 4.1).

As the heart begins to fail and cardiac output is reduced, there is a reduction in blood pressure; in compensation, there are several mechanisms that become active.

- Sympathetic nervous system
- Hormonal outflow (for example, adrenaline)
- Renin–angiotensin–aldosterone system

Table 4.1 Pathophysiological changes associated with heart failure

Pathophysiological changes	Description
Myocardial contractile dysfunction	The myocardium, the heart's muscular tissue, experiences diminished contractility. Reduction in the heart's ability to contract and pump blood efficiently results in a decreased cardiac output. Factors such as chronic ischaemia, inflammation or toxic exposures can contribute to contractile dysfunction.
Ventricular remodelling	Chronic pressure or volume overload can lead to ventricular remodelling. This occurs in response to increased stress. When this happens, the myocardium undergoes structural changes. The changes can include chamber dilation and hypertrophy. In the beginning, this remodelling is a compensatory mechanism to maintain cardiac output; however, over time, it becomes maladaptive.
Haemodynamic changes	
Heart failure is associated with significant haemodynamic alterations, which further complicates the condition:	
Increased afterload	Conditions such as hypertension increase the afterload, the resistance the heart must overcome to eject blood into the systemic circulation. In particular, the left ventricle must work harder against the elevated arterial pressure; this leads to hypertrophy and decreased contractility.
Volume overload	Volume overload occurs when the heart is exposed to an excessive volume of blood; this causes it to stretch and dilate. Often, this is seen in valvular disorders such as mitral regurgitation or aortic insufficiency. The dilated heart chambers are less efficient at pumping blood.
Neurohormonal activation	
As a response to reduced cardiac output, the body activates several neurohormonal mechanisms as compensation. Initially, these mechanisms help maintain blood pressure and perfusion. However, they become detrimental over time:	
Sympathetic nervous system activation	The sympathetic nervous system releases norepinephrine, which then increases heart rate and contractility. While these effects can initially support cardiac output, chronic sympathetic activation will then contribute to myocardial damage and arrhythmias.
Renin–angiotensin–aldosterone system (RAAS)	The RAAS is activated, leading to vasoconstriction and sodium and water retention. This mechanism increases intravascular volume, but prolonged activation can exacerbate congestion and further strain the heart.
Structural changes in the heart	
Chronic stress on the heart leads to structural changes, referred to collectively as cardiac remodelling. These changes include:	
Chamber dilation	The heart chambers, especially the left ventricle, may dilate to accommodate increased volume (see Figure 4.1). Initially, this dilation helps in maintaining stroke volume, but it eventually impairs contractility.
Hypertrophy	In response to pressure overload, the myocardium may undergo hypertrophy, thickening of the ventricular walls. This is an attempt to reduce wall stress, but it has the potential to compromise diastolic function and to increase oxygen demand.
Extracellular matrix alterations	Changes in the extracellular matrix composition can further impair cardiac function. Fibrosis, an excessive deposition of collagen fibres, can stiffen the myocardium and interfere with electrical conduction.

Source: Adapted from Nangle (2021); Schwinger (2021).

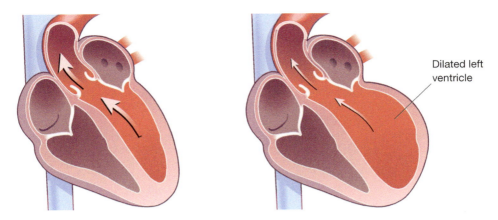

FIGURE 4.1   The structurally normal heart and the heart with an enlarged left ventricle

Activation of these mechanisms leads to an increase in total peripheral resistance, which has the short-term effect of increasing tissue perfusion. It also increases afterload and the work that the failing ventricle has to do, thereby exacerbating the original problem.

There are many different conditions leading to chronic heart failure, with possible overlap between categories. Causes (aetiology) are found in Box 4.1.

BOX 4.1   CAUSES OF HEART FAILURE

Myocardial disease:
- Coronary artery disease (most common)
- Hypertension.

Cardiomyopathies:
- Familial
- Infective
- Immune-mediated (such as autoimmune)
- Toxins (for example, alcohol or cocaine)
- Pregnancy
- Infiltrative (including, sarcoidosis, amyloidosis, haemochromatosis and connective tissue disease).

Valvular heart disease (for example, aortic stenosis)
Pericardial disease:
- Constrictive pericarditis
- Pericardial effusion

Congenital heart disease
Arrhythmias (for example, atrial fibrillation and other tachyarrythmias)
High output states:
- Anaemia
- Thyrotoxicosis

- Phaeochromocytoma
- Septicaemia
- Liver failure
- Arteriovenous shunts
- Paget's disease
- Thiamine (vitamin B1) deficiency

Volume overload:

- End-stage chronic kidney disease
- Nephrotic syndrome

Obesity

Drugs including:

- Alcohol
- Cocaine
- Non-steroidal anti-inflammatory drugs, beta-blockers and calcium-channel blockers may exacerbate pre-existing heart failure

Source: Adapted from Feather, Randall, and Waterhouse (2021) and British Medical Journal Best Practice (2024); Clare (2020).

Survival for those people with end-stage heart failure is poor. Regardless of the best possible medical management (including cardiac re-synchronisation therapy), only 65% of patients in New York Heart Association (NYHA) class IV are alive at an average follow-up of 17 months (BMJ Best Practice 2024).

Around 50% of people with heart failure will die within five years of diagnosis (Yancy et al. 2017; Taylor et al. 2019). Prognosis can be difficult to estimate or to state a prognosis for a person because heart failure often brings with it an unpredictable trajectory. The person may experience stable periods interrupted by episodic acute destabilisation. Poor prognostic indicators related to a poor prognosis can include:

- Increased age.
- Reduced ejection fraction (problems with heart's pumping action).
- The presence of comorbidities (for example, atrial fibrillation, chronic kidney disease, chronic obstructive pulmonary disease, depression and diabetes mellitus).
- Worsening severity of symptoms (based on the NYHA classification; see Table 4.4).
- The presence of signs that include raised jugular venous pressure, third heart sound, low systolic blood pressure and tachycardia.
- Obesity or cachexia.
- Smoking.
- Heart failure caused by ischaemic heart disease and specifically a history of MI.
- The presence of complex ventricular arrhythmias.

(BMJ Best Practice 2024; ESC 2021)

The complications associated with heart failure are outlined in Table 4.2.

Heart failure's pathophysiology is a multifaceted process involving impaired cardiac function, haemodynamic changes, neurohormonal activation and structural remodelling. The pathophysiological alterations collectively contribute to the clinical manifestations and progression of heart failure. It is important to understand these changes to diagnose and care for people and manage this complex syndrome in an effective and patient-centred way.

Table 4.2 Complications associated with heart failure

Complication	Discussion
Cardiac arrhythmias	Atrial fibrillation (see Box 4.2) is the most common arrhythmia in people with heart failure. The prevalence increases with age and the severity of heart failure.
	Ventricular arrhythmias are common in those with heart failure, particularly those with dilated left ventricle and reduced ejection fraction.
Depression	Major depressive disorder is present in up to 20% of people with heart failure.
Pleural effusion	Results from increasing pressure in the pleural cavities.
Cachexia (wasting)	Wasting occurs in lean tissue (muscle mass) and fat.
	Cachexia is associated with more severe symptoms, reduced functional capacity, more frequent hospitalisation and decreased survival rates.
Anaemia	People with heart failure will often have anaemia, which can worsen heart failure symptoms.
Chronic kidney disease (CKD)	CKD is common in people with heart failure with an impaired response to treatment with diuretics and angiotensin-converting enzyme inhibitors.
Acute kidney injury (AKI)	People with heart failure have a high risk of developing AKI either due to their low perfusion state or due to the medication used to treat heart failure.
Sexual dysfunction	Sexual dysfunction is common in people with heart failure. This may be related to cardiovascular disease, fatigue, weakness, the use of drugs (for example, beta-blockers) or depression and anxiety.
Sudden cardiac death	Around 30–40% of deaths in those with heart failure are related to sudden cardiac death.

Source: Adapted from Hagler et al. (2023), ESC (2021) and British Medical Journal Best Practice (2024).

BOX 4.2 ATRIAL FIBRILLATION

Atrial fibrillation is a common and potentially serious heart rhythm disorder, also known as an arrhythmia. In atrial fibrillation, the heart's upper chambers, the atria, quiver or fibrillate instead of contracting rhythmically. This irregular and chaotic electrical activity in the atria can disrupt the heart's normal rhythm and cause a range of symptoms and complications (see Figure 4.2).

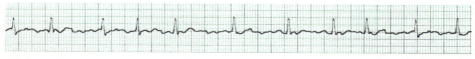

FIGURE 4.2 Atrial fibrillation

Atrial fibrillation is defined as when the atria are beating in an uncoordinated fashion, producing an irregularly irregular rhythm. This potentially dangerous rhythm may lead to emboli being transported into the aorta with subsequent migration up and into the cerebral blood vessels. This could result in stroke. This arrhythmia decreases the cardiac output by as much as 20–25%.

Source: Guerin and Mihaila (2021). With permission of John Wiley & Sons.

EPIDEMIOLOGY

The prevalence of heart failure is increasing, as a result of an ageing population and improved survival of chronic diseases contributing to heart failure (Clare 2020; Raleigh, Jefferies, and Wellings 2022). The prevalence of heart failure slowly increases with age until about 65 years of age; at that age it increases more rapidly. In the UK, the prevalence of heart failure is estimated to be about:

- 1 in 35 people 65–74 years of age.
- 1 in 15 people 75–84 years of age.
- Just over one in seven people 85 years of age or older (NICE 2018).

The British Heart Foundation (2023) estimates that around 690 000 people in the UK are registered with a general practitioner (GP) as having heart failure. It has been estimated that more than 900 000 people in the UK have heart failure with approximately 200 000 new diagnoses of heart failure annually. There are geographical variations in heart failure epidemiology across the UK and globally. Globally, there are around 64 million people affected worldwide (Savarese et al. 2023). Those with heart failure are two to three times more likely to have a stroke. Attempts to decrease the social and economic burden have become a major global public health priority.

Cardiovascular disease is among the largest contributors to health inequalities. Those people who live in England's most deprived areas will be four times more likely to die prematurely from cardiovascular disease than those living in the least deprived areas.

The National Health Service, public health services as well as local authorities must work together to address the wider determinants of health and inequalities, to reduce behavioural risk factors and to strengthen the prevention and early detection of heart failure (Raleigh, Jefferies, and Wellings 2022).

RISK FACTORS

There are many things that can increase the risk of heart failure. Some of those things are modifiable, for example, lifestyle habits; many others, however, are non-modifiable (out of the control of the individual) and these include age or ethnicity. The risk of heart failure increases if the person has one or more of the issues listed in Table 4.3.

Heart failure is common in both men and women, though men often develop heart failure at a younger age than women will. Women more commonly have HFpEF (when the heart does not fill with enough blood). Men are more likely to have HFrEF (when the left ventricle is not squeezing effectively). Women may have worse symptoms than men.

Table 4.3 Risk of heart failure increases if the person has one or more of the issues listed

Factor	Discussion
Ageing	People 65 years or older have a higher risk of heart failure. Older adults are also more likely to have other health conditions causing heart failure (see Box 4.3).
Family history of heart failure	This makes the risk of heart failure higher. Genetics may also play a role. Some changes or mutations to genes may make heart tissue weaker or less flexible.
Unhealthy lifestyle habits	For example, an unhealthy diet, smoking, using cocaine or other illicit drugs, heavy alcohol use and lack of physical activity increase the risk of heart failure.
Heart or blood vessel conditions, serious lung disease or infections such as human immunodeficiency virus or COVID-19	These conditions raise the risk. This is also true for long-term health conditions such as obesity, high blood pressure, diabetes, sleep apnoea, chronic kidney disease, anaemia, thyroid disease or iron overload (haemochromatosis). Cancer treatments such as radiation and chemotherapy can injure the heart and increase risk as well. Atrial fibrillation, a common type of irregular heart rhythm, can also cause heart failure.
Black Caribbean, Black African and Black Other groups	More likely to have heart failure than people of other races. Often these patients have more serious cases of heart failure and experience heart failure at a younger age.
Living in an area of high deprivation	There is a higher prevalence in deprived communities, reflecting the higher prevalence of risk factors among those communities.

Source: Adapted from Raleigh, Jefferies, and Wellings (2022); National Heart, Lung, and Blood Institute (2022).

BOX 4.3 HEART FAILURE CHANGES WITH AGEING

Age-related changes in the heart and cardiovascular system increase the risk of heart failure. Interstitial collagen within the myocardium increases, which causes the myocardium to stiffen and myocardial relaxation is then prolonged. These changes lead to a significant reduction in diastolic left ventricular function, even in healthy older people. There is a modest decline in systolic function occurring with ageing. An age-related decrease in myocardial and vascular responsiveness to beta-adrenergic stimulation can further impair the ability of the cardiovascular system to give an effective response to increased work demands.

It is essential to recognise that while ageing is a significant risk factor for heart failure, it is not an inevitable consequence of getting older. There are many older individuals who maintain excellent heart health through a combination of healthy lifestyle choices, regular medical check-ups and appropriate management of chronic conditions. Early detection and proactive management of risk factors can help to reduce the risk and the severity of heart failure in older adults.

Understanding the risk factors associated with heart failure and the population groups who show distinct risk factor trend differences can help in designing contemporary tailored prevention programmes (Lawson et al. 2020).

CLINICAL PRESENTATION

Chronic heart failure can be difficult to diagnose because the symptoms and signs are often non-specific. Manifestations of heart failure differ depending on the extent to which the left ventricle and the right ventricle are initially affected. Clinical severity varies significantly and is usually classified according to the NYHA system (Brennan 2018) (see Table 4.4).

Table 4.4 Classification of the severity of heart failure based on the New York Heart Association functional classification

Class	Description
Class I (mild)	There is no limitation on physical activity. Regular physical activity does not cause undue fatigue, palpitations or dyspnoea. Heart failure is essentially well treated.
Class II (mild)	Slight limitations of physical activity are apparent. The person is comfortable at rest however; regular physical activity results in fatigue, palpitation or dyspnoea.
Class III (moderate)	There is a marked limitation of physical activity. The person is comfortable at rest; less than ordinary activity, however, will cause fatigue, palpitation or dyspnoea.
Class IV (severe)	The person is unable to carry out any physical activity without experiencing discomfort. There are symptoms of cardiac failure at rest. Essentially, the patient is housebound.

Source: Adapted from Clare (2020); Brennan (2018).

The examples of ordinary activity cited in Table 4.4 may be modified for older, debilitated patients.

SIGNS AND SYMPTOMS OF RIGHT-SIDED HEART FAILURE

Pitting oedema may be observed in the sacral area of a patient confined to bed, as well as on the feet and legs when the patient is sitting (see Box 4.4). This is due to the impaired pumping ability of the heart, and as a result, fluid accumulates in the tissues, resulting in weight gain.

BOX 4.4   PERIPHERAL OEDEMA

Ageing often leads to damage to the skin integrity and reduced healing. This is exacerbated by the presence of peripheral oedema making the skin more susceptible to damage and tears as the skin is stretched by the swelling tissues. Oedematous legs are heavier; the patient may drag their legs across the bed or chair, leading to shearing forces that could break the skin. Oedematous skin is more friable and less resistant to damage that could be caused by knocks and minor impacts, leading to an increase in the incidence of broken skin. The associated reduction in healing increases the potential for leg ulcers to develop.

Caring for a patient with leg oedema in any setting is an opportunity to achieve outcomes associated with assessing skin and/or risk assessment. For instance, the patient's bedside environment or home should be checked for unnecessary equipment that may lead to bumps and scrapes and the skin should be assessed for rashes or sores when removing compression stockings.

Source: Clare (2020). With permission of John Wiley & Sons.

Enlargement of the organs such as the liver (hepatomegaly) and the spleen (splenomegaly) can cause pressure on the surrounding organs such as the stomach.

Pleural effusion may occur due to increased capillary pressure.

Distended jugular veins are a visible sign in those patients who experience right-sided heart failure.

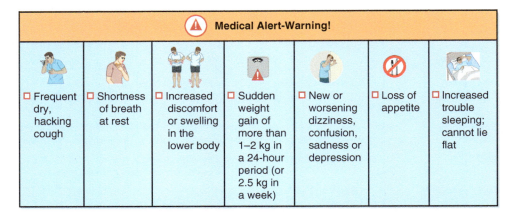

FIGURE 4.3   Red flags for heart failure

Patients may have difficulty in breathing (dyspnoea). Dyspnoea can occur when the patient exerts themselves or lies down (orthopnoea). They may become severely short of breath. There may be a persistent cough or wheezing with white or pink blood-tinged sputum (haemoptysis). Breathing may be rapid, shallow breathing (tachypnoea).

There may be nausea and anorexia and the patient may be fatigued. Nausea and anorexia can exacerbate the overall condition in heart failure patients, and inadequate nutrition can weaken the body and worsen symptoms.

Jaundice and coagulation problems may be present as a result of liver damage.

Red flags associated with heart failure can be found in Figure 4.3.

SIGNS AND SYMPTOMS OF LEFT-SIDED HEART FAILURE

Patients with left-sided heart failure may develop dyspnoea in the early stages as a result of fluid accumulation in the pulmonary capillary bed, which results in poor exchange of gases (oxygen and carbon dioxide) in the lungs.

Dizziness, fatigue and weakness are due to the poor oxygenation of the body tissues, resulting from low cardiac output and oxygen saturation. Reduced oxygen supply to the brain may cause dizziness, disorientation, confusion and unconsciousness.

Orthopnoea, peripheral oedema and productive cough with frothy sputum may be present. The patient may be wheezing as a result of bronchospasm. There can be crackles at the lung bases due to pulmonary oedema when the lungs are auscultated.

Tachycardia can accompany respiratory problems. Cyanosis, the bluish discolouration of the mucous membranes around the lips and in the nail bed, may be present.

Figure 4.4 illustrates some of the signs and symptoms associated with heart failure.

CLINICAL INVESTIGATIONS AND DIAGNOSIS

Diagnosing heart failure typically involves a combination of medical history assessment, physical examination and various tests and imaging studies. National Institute for Health and Care Excellence (2018) suggests a careful and detailed history is obtained, clinical examination is performed and tests are carried out to confirm the presence of heart failure.

Clinical Investigations and Diagnosis 71

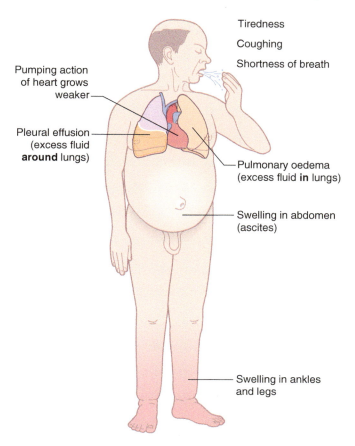

FIGURE 4.4   Some of the signs and symptoms associated with heart failure

Heart failure is diagnosed when:

1. There are symptoms of heart failure (at rest or on exertion).
2. There is objective evidence of cardiac dysfunction.
3. There is a response to treatment for heart failure.

For heart failure to be diagnosed, at least Points 1 and 2 must be met, as the signs and symptoms of other disease processes (such as pulmonary disease) can be similar to the early stages of heart failure (Clare 2020).

The tests and investigations undertaken include (European Society of Cardiology 2021):

- Echocardiography, to assess heart function and the heart valves.
- Cardiac radionuclide scan (also known as a nuclear cardiology scan or myocardial perfusion imaging), a medical imaging test used to assess the blood flow to the heart muscle and detect areas of reduced blood supply or ischaemia.
- MRI scan.

- Blood tests for:
  - Electrolytes
  - Albumin
  - Creatinine
  - B-type natriuretic peptide (BNP) or N-terminal pro-B-type natriuretic peptide (NT-proBNP).
- A 12-lead electrocardiogram to assess for heart disease.
- Cardiac catheterisation to assess for heart disease and assess heart function.
- Chest X-ray to assess the heart size and for signs of pulmonary oedema.
- Exercise tolerance test to assess for heart disease and exercise ability (if appropriate).

MANAGEMENT

A multidisciplinary team approach is advocated. The heart failure team should be a representative of the expertise of a range of professionals who are based in the hospital or in the community and this will include:

- Cardiologists
- GPs
- Care of the elderly physicians
- Heart failure specialist nurses
- Palliative care nurses
- Pharmacists
- Psychologists

The transition between hospital and home following admission for an episode of acute heart failure is a period of concern, which can be characterised by poor communication between healthcare professionals involved with inpatient and community care. Patients and their caregivers may feel discharge is sudden and unexpected and as a result, may feel ill-prepared.

The provision of seamless transitions with the hospital setting and in the community requires a number of strategies to be employed, including a structured discharge plan shared with the patient and those involved in their care. This includes the provision of educational materials and interventions to enhance communication between different health, care and voluntary sectors.

Treatment of heart failure includes the administration of medications, for example, diuretics, angiotensin-converting enzyme (ACE) inhibitors and beta-blockers. Pharmacological approaches to managing patients with chronic heart failure are aimed at reducing their risk for death, relieving symptoms, improving exercise tolerance and reducing the incidence of acute exacerbations, e.g. pulmonary oedema (Guerin and Mihaila 2021; Lainscak et al. 2015). Medications used in heart failure aim to:

- Control excessive fluid: diuretics.

- Reduce the heart's workload: calcium channel blockers, angiotensin II receptor blockers, ACE inhibitors, amiodarone, beta-1 blockers and anticoagulants.
- Optimise the contractility of the heart: digoxin and nitrates.

Patients hospitalised with severe heart failure may require treatment with inotropic sympathomimetics, such as dopamine or dobutamine. These drugs create the same response as sympathetic nervous system activation; they increase the force of contraction of the ventricles and increase heart rate. Patients receiving these drugs should be cared for in a high-dependency unit or coronary care unit and will require continuous cardiac monitoring and hourly blood pressure measurement.

Furthermore, as the patient will be administered diuretic therapy and may have their fluids restricted, strict fluid balance monitoring will be required.

Patients should be cared for in an upright or semi-recumbent position (at the angle the patient finds most comfortable) and oxygen therapy administered, as prescribed. The combination of shortness of breath (including rapid mouth breathing) and oxygen therapy will result in a dry mouth and regular mouth care should be offered, as well as the provision of humidified oxygen.

Peripheral oedema along with shortness of breath and lethargy increase the risk of pressure sores and pressure area care is essential.

END OF LIFE CARE

Dying patients can have needs that will differ from those of other patients. For their needs to be met, dying patients must first be identified. Patients with heart failure at the end of life may experience progressive functional decline, an extended indefinite period of severe dysfunction. Heart failure may not be steadily progressive; rather, functional ability can decrease irregularly due to periodic and sometimes unpredictable acute exacerbations of the underlying disorder.

The principles of end of life care should be based on sensitive communication about what to expect. This will include a discussion regarding the uncertainty of prognosis and how care and treatment will be managed (Gleton and Larkin 2015). All patients and family members should be taught about disease progression and the risk of sudden cardiac death. For some patients, it is improving the quality of life that is just as important as increasing the quantity of life. Therefore, it is important to determine patients' wishes about cardiopulmonary resuscitation if their condition deteriorates, especially when the heart failure is already at an advanced stage.

Reassurance should be given that symptoms will be relieved, and they should be encouraged to seek medical attention early if there is a significant change in symptoms. A multidisciplinary team approach is required, including pharmacists, nurses, social workers and, if required, a spiritual healthcare team.

HEALTH TEACHING

It is important to remember many people with heart failure lead full, enjoyable lives. Also, it should also be noted not all heart failure is the same and no two patients are the same; as such, a tailored approach to health education and promotion is needed.

A diagnosis of heart failure can be worrying for patients and their families. It can raise concerns about what the patient can and cannot do as well as what the future is going to be like.

Learning how to manage symptoms and medication can help the person to keep the condition under control. The British Heart Foundation suggests five ways to manage heart failure:

1. Take your medications (if you think you are experiencing side effects, talk to the nurse specialist or doctor).
2. Keep as active as you can (if doing something makes you feel unwell, then avoid doing it).
3. Report new or worsening symptoms to the GP, doctor, heart failure nurse or community nurse (when earlier action is taken the better the outcome).
4. Weigh yourself every day before you eat or drink (even an increase of 1 kg can be significant; it may mean excess fluid is building up).
5. Avoid excessive salt (too much salt can increase blood pressure).

Make sure the person is offered an annual influenza vaccine and a once-only pneumococcal vaccination. Consider referral to smoking cessation services and offer advice that those with heart failure should not drink alcohol beyond the recommended levels.

Ensure referral is made to a supervised exercise-based rehabilitation programme. Those with stable heart failure may engage in normal sexual activity that does not provoke undue symptoms.

It is the person's responsibility to inform the Driver and Vehicle Licensing Agency of any condition that may affect their ability to drive and people should check with their insurer that they are still covered to drive (see Assessing fitness to drive: a guide for medical professionals – GOV.UK [www.gov.uk]).

General advice with regard to travel includes:

- To continue regular medication, carry extra medication as a precaution during travel.
- For aeroplane travel, carry medication in hand luggage.
- Carry a written record of medical history and current drug treatment.
- To monitor fluid intake and risk of dehydration, for example, during a flight and in hot climates.
- To be aware of potential adverse reactions to sun exposure with certain drugs (for example, amiodarone).

The Civil Aviation Authority provides information regarding fitness for flying can be obtained here:

Assessing fitness to fly: Guidelines for health professionals (www.caa.co.uk)

CONCLUSION

Heart failure is a complex, chronic condition that requires a comprehensive understanding of its pathophysiology, clinical manifestations and management strategies. Recognising the signs and symptoms of heart failure early is critical to improving patient outcomes. Effective management includes not only pharmacological interventions but also lifestyle modifications, patient education, psychological support for the patient and their family and ongoing monitoring.

Understanding the various types of heart failure allows for tailored care approaches that address the specific needs of each patient. Emphasising patient-centred care plays a pivotal role in coordinating multidisciplinary efforts, advising and informing patients about self-management and providing them with emotional support.

Staying informed about the latest evidence-based practices and fostering a compassionate approach to care can make a profound difference in the lives of patients living with heart failure.

GLOSSARY OF TERMS

Afterload: The resistance the heart must overcome to eject blood into the circulatory system, affected by blood pressure and vascular resistance.

Angiotensin-converting enzyme (ACE) inhibitors: Medications dilating blood vessels and reducing the heart's workload.

Atherosclerosis: Build-up of plaque (cholesterol and other substances) in the arteries, narrowing blood vessels and reducing blood flow.

Beta-blockers: Medications blocking the effects of adrenaline on the heart, reducing heart rate and blood pressure.

B-type natriuretic peptide (BNP): A hormone released by the heart in response to increased pressure, often elevated in heart failure and used for diagnosis.

Cardiac output (CO): The amount of blood pumped by the heart in one minute, an important measure of heart function.

Cardiomegaly: Enlargement of the heart, often seen on chest X-rays in heart failure.

Diuretics: Medications promoting the removal of excess fluid and sodium from the body, reducing oedema.

Dyspnoea: Difficulty breathing.

Ejection fraction (EF): The percentage of blood ejected from the left ventricle with each heartbeat, used to assess the heart's pumping function.

Heart failure: A chronic condition in which the heart cannot pump blood effectively, leading to insufficient oxygen and nutrient delivery to the body's tissues.

Left ventricular failure: Heart failure primarily affecting the left ventricle, leading to reduced blood flow to the body.

Oedema: Swelling caused by the accumulation of excess fluid in the body's tissues, often seen in heart failure patients.

Orthopnoea: Difficulty breathing when lying flat, often relieved by sitting up or elevating the head.

Paroxysmal nocturnal dyspnoea: Sudden severe shortness of breath that awakens a person during the night.

Preload: The amount of blood returning to the heart before each contraction, influencing the heart's stretching and subsequent pumping.

Pulmonary oedema: Accumulation of fluid in the lungs, leading to symptoms such as shortness of breath and coughing.

Right ventricular failure: Heart failure primarily affecting the right ventricle, causing blood to back up into the veins and peripheral tissues.

MULTIPLE CHOICE QUESTIONS

1. What is heart failure?
   a) A heart condition characterised by an enlarged heart
   b) A sudden loss of heart function
   c) A condition in which the heart cannot pump blood effectively
   d) A condition where the heart beats too slowly

2. Which of the following is NOT a common symptom of heart failure?
   a) Shortness of breath
   b) Swelling of the ankles and legs
   c) Persistent cough
   d) Increased energy levels

3. What is the hallmark symptom of right-sided heart failure?
   a) Fatigue
   b) Shortness of breath
   c) Peripheral oedema
   d) Chest pain

4. What is the most common cause of right-sided heart failure?
   a) Coronary artery disease
   b) Hypertension
   c) Pulmonary hypertension
   d) Valvular heart disease

5. What is an ejection fraction?
   a) The amount of blood pumped by the heart with each beat
   b) The volume of blood remaining in the heart after each beat
   c) The percentage of blood ejected from the heart's left ventricle
   d) The pressure in the heart's chambers during systole

6. Which diagnostic test is used to measure ejection fraction?
   a) Electrocardiogram (ECG)
   b) Chest X-ray
   c) Echocardiogram
   d) Blood pressure measurement

7. Which class of medications is commonly used to manage heart failure and reduce fluid retention?
   a) Beta-blockers
   b) Angiotensin-converting enzyme (ACE) inhibitors
   c) Diuretics
   d) Anticoagulants

8. What is the primary goal of treatment for heart failure?
   a) To cure the condition
   b) To improve ejection fraction
   c) To relieve symptoms, improve quality of life and reduce hospitalisations
   d) To reduce blood pressure

9. Which lifestyle modification is essential for managing heart failure?
   a) Smoking cessation
   b) Avoiding physical activity
   c) Consuming a high-sodium diet
   d) Skipping medications

10. What is orthopnoea?
    a) Difficulty swallowing
    b) Difficulty breathing when lying flat
    c) Irregular heart rhythm
    d) Chest pain

REFERENCES

British Heart Foundation. (2023). *UK Factsheet.* BHF UK CVD factsheet. https://www.bhf.org.uk/-/media/files/for-professionals/research/heart-statistics/bhf-cvd-statistics-uk-factsheet.pdf?rev=c64051a5b118450490f48b1e5b72f1ff&hash=D4DAD77307F06B5883373456597729A6 (accessed September 2023).

British Medical Journal Best Practice (2024) *Chronic congestive heart failure.* BMJ Publishing. Heart failure with reduced ejection fraction – Symptoms, diagnosis and treatment. https://bestpractice.bmj.com/topics/en-gb/61.

Brennan, E.J. (2018). Chronic heart failure nursing: integrated multidisciplinary care. *British Journal of Nursing* 27 (12): 681–688.

Clare, C. (2020). The person with a cardiovascular disorder (Chapter 25). In: *Nursing Practice, Knowledge and Care,* 3e (eds. I. Peate and A. Mitchell). Oxford: Wiley.

European Society of Cardiology. (2021). 2021 ESC guidelines for the diagnosis and treatment of acute and chronic heart failure. *European Heart Journal* 42 (36): 3599–3726. doi:10.1093/eurheartj/ehab368

Feather, A., Randall, D., and Waterhouse, M. (2021). *Kumar and Clark's Clinical Medicine*, 10e. London: Elsevier.

Gleton, C. and Larkin, P.J. (eds.) (2015). *Palliative Care Nursing at a Glance.* Oxford: Wiley.

Guerin, J. and Mihaila, C. (2021). Medications used in the cardiovascular system (Chapter 10). In: *Fundamentals Pharmacology* (eds. I. Peate and B. Hill). Oxford: Wiley.

Hagler, D., Harding, M.M., Kwang, J. et al. (2023). *Lewis's Medical-Surgical Nursing,* 12e. St Louis: Elsevier.

Lainscak, M., Pelliccia, F., Rosano, G. et al. (2015). Safety profile of mineralocorticoid receptor antagonists: spironolactone and eplerenone. *International Journal of Cardiology* 200: 25–29.

Lawson, A., Zaccardi, F., Squire, I. et al. (2020). Risk factors for heart failure: 20-year population-based trends by sex, socioeconomic status, and ethnicity. *Circulation: Heart Failure* 13 (2): e006472. doi.org/10.1161/CIRCHEARTFAILURE.119.006472.

Nangle, V. (2021). The heart and associate disorders (Chapter 8). In: *Fundamentals of Applied Pathophysiology,* 4e (ed. I. Peate). Oxford: Wiley.

National Heart, Lung, and Blood Institute. (2022). *Heart Failure. Causes and Risk Factors.* https://www.nhlbi.nih.gov/health/heart-failure/causes (accessed October 2023).

National Institute for Health and Care Excellence. (2018). Chronic heart failure in adults: diagnosis and management. https://www.nice.org.uk/guidance/ng106 (accessed September 2023).

Raleigh, V., Jefferies, D., and Wellings, D. (2022). Cardiovascular disease in England: supporting leaders to take action. https://www.kingsfund.org.uk/insight-and-analysis/reports/cardiovascular-disease-england (accessed September 2023).

Schwinger, R.H.G. (2021). Pathophysiology of heart failure. *Cardiovascular Diagnosis and Therapy* 11 (1): 263–276. doi:10.21037/cdt-20-302.

Savarese, G., Moritz-Becher, P., Lund, L.H. et al. (2023). Global burden of heart failure: a comprehensive and updated review of epidemiology. *Cardiovascular Research* 118 (17): 3272–3287. doi:10.1093/cvr/cvac013.

Taylor, C.J., Ordóñez-Mena, J.M., Roalfe, A.K. et al. (2019). Trends in survival after a diagnosis of heart failure in the United Kingdom 2000–2017: population based cohort study. *British Medical Journal (Clinical Research Edition)* 367. https://pubmed.ncbi.nlm.nih.gov/30760447 (accessed October 2023).

Yancy, C.W., Jessup, M., Bozkurt, B. et al. (2017). 2017 ACC/AHA/HFSA focused update of the 2013 ACCF/AHA guideline for the management of heart failure: a report of the American College of Cardiology/American Heart Association task force on clinical practice guidelines and the Heart Failure Society of America. https://pubmed.ncbi.nlm.nih.gov/28455343 (accessed October 2023).

Cardiogenic Shock CHAPTER 5

Cardiogenic shock is also known as cardiac shock; it happens when the heart is unable to pump sufficient blood and oxygen to the brain and other vital organs. This is a life-threatening emergency and is treatable if diagnosed right away. This critical medical condition is typically caused by a primary cardiac dysfunction. Understanding the pathophysiology of cardiogenic shock is crucial for healthcare professionals, as it forms the basis for appropriate assessment and management of this life-threatening condition.

This chapter begins with a discussion on cardiac arrest. Discussing cardiac arrest and cardiogenic shock together is important as they are closely related medical conditions that often occur in sequence or as a result of one another. Understanding the connection between these two conditions is crucial for healthcare professionals and can have a significant impact on patient care and outcomes.

CARDIAC ARREST

Cardiac arrest is a sudden state of circulatory failure due to a loss of cardiac systolic function. Cardiac mechanical activity ceases, resulting in the absence of circulating blood flow. Cardiac arrest impedes blood from flowing to vital organs; this deprives them of oxygen. If left untreated, this results in death. Sudden cardiac arrest is the unexpected cessation of circulation within a short period of symptom onset (often without warning).

A heart attack is not the same as a cardiac arrest. A heart attack occurs when one of the coronary arteries becomes blocked. The myocardium does not receive its critical blood supply, and if this is left untreated, the myocardium will begin to deteriorate as it fails to receive enough oxygen. A cardiac arrest occurs when a person's heart stops pumping blood around the body, and they stop breathing normally. In adults, a number of cardiac arrests occur because of a heart attack as a person having a heart attack may develop a dangerous arrhythmia, which can cause cardiac arrest. A heart attack and a cardiac arrest are both emergency situations, and help must be summoned immediately.

In adults, sudden cardiac arrest results principally from cardiac disease. In a significant percentage of patients, it is sudden cardiac arrest that is the first manifestation of heart disease. Other causes include circulatory shock due to non-cardiac disorders (such as pulmonary embolism, gastrointestinal haemorrhage or trauma), ventilatory failure and metabolic disturbance (this includes drug overdose) (Tsao et al. 2023).

Cardiac arrest causes global ischaemia, bringing with it consequences at the cellular level that adversely affect organ function even after resuscitation and restoration of perfusion. The main consequences involve direct cellular damage and oedema formation. Cerebral oedema is particularly harmful because there is minimal room within the cranium for the brain to expand; often this results in increased intracranial pressure along with a corresponding decreased cerebral perfusion post-resuscitation. A significant proportion of patients who have been successfully resuscitated will have short- or long-term cerebral dysfunction that is manifested by altered alertness (from mild confusion to coma), seizures or both.

EPIDEMIOLOGY: CARDIAC ARREST

Epidemiology plays a pivotal role in cardiac arrest management by providing essential information (data) on incidence, risk factors, outcomes and the impact of interventions. This knowledge informs healthcare policy, public health initiatives and clinical practice guidelines, ultimately contributing to improved cardiac arrest prevention, response and patient outcomes. Key information on the epidemiology and outcome of out-of-hospital and in-hospital cardiac arrest are presented in Table 5.1.

Table 5.1 Epidemiology of cardiac arrest

Out-of-hospital cardiac arrest (OHCA) in the UK	• Annually, National Health Service (NHS) Ambulance Services attempt resuscitation in approximately 30 000 people. • The incidence of OHCA is approximately 55 per 100 000 inhabitants each year. • Most cardiac arrests (72%) occur in the home or the workplace (15%). • Half of all OHCA are witnessed by a bystander. • Most cardiac arrests occur in adults (98%); one-third (33%) of those were aged 15–64 years. • Eight of 10 OHCA are due to a cardiac cause. • In 7 of 10 OHCA, bystander cardiopulmonary resuscitation (CPR) is attempted. • Public access defibrillator use is reported as being used in less than 1 in 10 OHCA. • The initial rhythm is shockable in approximately one in four OHCA (22–25%). • A return of spontaneous circulation (ROSC) is achieved in approximately 30% of attempted resuscitations. • When resuscitation is attempted, just fewer than 1 in 10 (9%) people survive to hospital discharge following OHCA.
In-hospital cardiac arrest (IHCA) in the UK	• The annual incidence of in-hospital cardiac arrest (IHCA) is 1 to 1.5 per 1000 hospital admissions. • The average age of those sustaining an IHCA is 70 years. A quarter (26.7%) are aged 16–64 years. • Most cardiac arrests (85%) occur onwards and in patients admitted to hospital for medical reasons. • The initial rhythm is shockable in 17% of cardiac arrests, pulseless electrical activity 52%, asystole 20% and the remainder are unknown or undetermined. • ROSC is achieved in half (53%) of those who are treated by a hospital's resuscitation team for IHCA. • A quarter (23.6%) of those treated by a hospital's resuscitation team for IHCA survive to hospital discharge. • More than four of five (83%) who survive hospital discharge have a favourable neurological outcome.

Source: Adapted from Perkins et al. (2021a).

RISK FACTORS ASSOCIATED WITH CARDIAC ARREST

Understanding the risk factors associated with cardiac arrest is vital for prevention, early detection, targeted interventions, resource allocation, research and public health efforts (see Box 5.1). By identifying and addressing these risk factors, healthcare professionals and public health organisations can work towards reducing the incidence and improving outcomes of cardiac arrest, ultimately saving lives.

BOX 5.1   RISK FACTORS ASSOCIATED WITH CARDIAC ARREST

- Coronary artery disease.
- Left ventricular dysfunction.
- Hypertrophic cardiomyopathy.
- Arrhythmogenic right ventricular dysplasia (a rare and inherited heart condition).
- Long QT syndrome, a rare and potentially life-threatening heart rhythm disorder.
- Medical or surgical emergency (such as pulmonary embolism, tension pneumothorax and drug toxicity).
- Illicit substance use (for example, opioid-induced respiratory depression leading to hypoxia-induced cardiac arrest, and stimulants, such as cocaine or amphetamines, can result in arrhythmia or ischaemia leading to cardiac arrest).

Other risk factors may include:

- Valvular heart disease
- Smoking
- Eating disorder or malnutrition
- Inherited syndromes of conduction abnormality (e.g. Brugada syndrome)

Source: Adapted from British Medical Journal Best Practice (2022).

GUIDELINES FOR ADULT BASIC LIFE SUPPORT

Cardiac arrest recognition is a key priority; it is the first step in initiating the emergency response to cardiac arrest. Box 5.2 outlines guidelines for adult basic life support.

BOX 5.2   ADULT BASIC LIFE SUPPORT GUIDELINES

Commence cardiopulmonary resuscitation (CPR)

- Ensure it is safe to approach the person.
- Commence CPR on an unresponsive person with absent or abnormal breathing.
- Agonal breathing should be considered a sign of cardiac arrest.

(Continued)

BOX 5.2 (CONTINUED)

- A short period of seizure-like movements may occur at the start of cardiac arrest. Assess the person after the seizure has stopped: if unresponsive and with absent or abnormal breathing, commence CPR.

Alert emergency services

- A lone bystander with a mobile phone should call 999, activate the speaker or another hands-free option and immediately start CPR, assisted by the dispatcher.
- If you are a lone rescuer, and you have to leave a victim to call the ambulance service, first alert the ambulance service and then commence CPR.

High-quality chest compressions

- Begin chest compressions as soon as possible.
- Deliver compressions on the lower half of the sternum.
- Compress to a depth of at least 5 cm but not more than 6 cm.
- Compress the chest at a rate of 100–120 per minute with as few interruptions as possible.
- Allow the chest to recoil completely after each compression; do not lean on the chest.
- Whenever feasible, carry out chest compressions on a firm surface.

Rescue breaths

- If you are trained to do so, after 30 compressions, provide two rescue breaths.
- Alternate between providing 30 compressions and two rescue breaths.
- If unable or unwilling to provide ventilation, give continuous chest compressions.

Automated electronic defibrillator (AED)

How to locate an AED

- The location of an AED should be indicated by clear signage.
- Ambulance services have available up-to-date information on defibrillator locations. A number of apps are available that list defibrillator locations.

When and how to use an AED

- As soon as the AED arrives, or if already available, switch it on.
- Attach electrode pads to the person's bare chest according to the position shown on the AED or on the pads.
- If more than one rescuer is present, continue CPR while pads are being attached.
- Follow the spoken (and/or visual) prompts from the AED.
- Ensure nobody is touching the person whilst the AED is analysing the heart rhythm.
- If a shock is indicated, ensure that nobody is touching the person. Push the shock button as prompted. Immediately restart CPR with 30 compressions. If no shock is indicated, immediately restart CPR with 30 compressions.
- In either case, continue with CPR as prompted by the AED. There will be a period of CPR (usually two minutes) before the AED prompts a further pause in CPR for rhythm analysis.

Shock 83

Compressions before defibrillation
- Continue CPR until an AED arrives and is switched on and attached to the person.
- Do not delay defibrillation to provide additional CPR once the defibrillator is ready.

Safety
- Ensure you, the person and bystanders are safe.
- Members of the public should start CPR for presumed cardiac arrest without concerns of causing harm to those not in cardiac arrest.
- Members of the public may safely perform chest compressions and use an AED risk of infection during compressions and harm from accidental shock during AED use is very low.

Foreign body airway obstruction
- Suspect choking if someone is suddenly unable to speak or talk, particularly if eating.
- Encourage the person to cough.
- If the cough becomes ineffective, give up to five back blows:
  - Lean the person forward.
  - Apply blows between shoulder blades using the heel of one hand.
- If back blows are ineffective, give up to five abdominal thrusts:
  - Stand behind the person, put both your arms around the upper part of their abdomen.
  - Lean the person forwards.
  - Clench your fist and place it between the umbilicus and ribcage.
  - Grasp your fist with the other hand and pull sharply inwards and upwards.
- If choking has not been relieved after five abdominal thrusts, continue alternating five back blows with five abdominal thrusts until it is relieved or the person becomes unresponsive.
- If the person becomes unresponsive, commence CPR.

Recovery position
For those with a decreased level of responsiveness due to medical illness or non-physical trauma, who do not meet the criteria for the initiation of rescue breathing or chest compressions (CPR), Resuscitation Council UK (RCUK) recommends they are placed into a lateral, side-lying recovery position.

Source: Adapted from Perkins et al. (2021b).

Figure 5.1 offers a flowchart that details the sequence of basic adult life support.

SHOCK

Shock is a state of organ hypoperfusion that results in cellular dysfunction and death. Mechanisms may involve decreased circulating volume, decreased cardiac output and vasodilation. Shock is a life-threatening condition characterised by a systemic failure of the body's circulatory system to provide adequate oxygen and nutrients to vital organs and tissues. The pathophysiological changes associated with shock can vary depending on the type of shock (see Table 5.2).

84 CHAPTER 5 Cardiogenic Shock

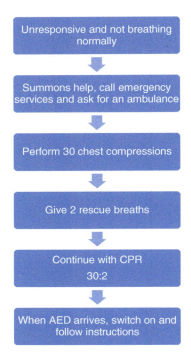

FIGURE 5.1 The sequence of basic adult life support. *Source:* Chadick (2021). With permission of John Wiley & Sons.

Table 5.2 Types of shock

Types of shock	Discussion
Hypovolaemic shock (a low circulating volume)	Hypovolaemic shock is caused by a significant decrease in intravascular volume. Diminished venous return (preload) results in decreased ventricular filling along with reduced stroke volume. Unless this is compensated for by increased heart rate, then cardiac output decreases.
	A common cause of this type of shock is bleeding (haemorrhagic shock), usually due to trauma, surgical interventions, peptic ulcer, oesophageal varices or ruptured aortic aneurysm. Bleeding may be overt, for example, haematemesis, melaena or concealed, such as ruptured ectopic pregnancy.
Distributive shock (vasodilation)	Distributive shock results from a relative reduction of intravascular volume caused by arterial or venous vasodilation; circulating blood volume is normal. In other situations, blood pools and cardiac output falls. Can be caused by: • Anaphylaxis (anaphylactic shock) • Bacterial infection with endotoxin release (septic shock) or exotoxin release (toxic shock) • Severe injury to the spinal cord, usually above T4 (neurogenic shock) • Ingestion of certain drugs or poisons, such as nitrates, opioids and adrenergic blockers
	Anaphylactic shock and septic shock often have a component of hypovolaemia as well.

Types of shock	Discussion
Cardiogenic shock	A relative or absolute reduction in cardiac output due to a primary cardiac disorder. Obstructive shock is caused by mechanical factors that interfere with filling or emptying of the heart or great vessels. There is a primary decrease in cardiac output (this also includes distributive shock).

All types of shock, however, share some common features. What follows is a brief outline of the general pathophysiological changes that are associated with shock.

Hypoperfusion: Shock is primarily defined by inadequate tissue perfusion, where there is an insufficient supply of oxygen and nutrients to meet the metabolic demands of the body's cells. This leads to cellular hypoxia (oxygen deprivation) and it can affect various organs and tissues.

Cellular hypoxia: Reduced oxygen delivery to cells; this triggers a cascade of cellular changes, including impaired ATP (adenosine triphosphate) production, the primary energy source for cells. As ATP levels decrease, cellular functions become compromised, leading to a breakdown in normal cellular metabolism.

Lactic acidosis: When there is sufficient oxygen for aerobic metabolism, cells switch to anaerobic metabolism. This produces lactic acid as a byproduct. The accumulation of lactic acid in the bloodstream leads to metabolic acidosis, contributing to further tissue dysfunction.

Activation of the stress response: The body responds to shock by initiating the stress response. This involves the release of stress hormones, for example, adrenaline and cortisol. These hormones increase heart rate, vasoconstriction and myocardial contractility, all aimed at improving oxygen delivery to vital organs.

Cardiovascular changes: Shock often leads to alterations in the cardiovascular system, including:

- Hypotension: A key feature of shock is low blood pressure, resulting from reduced cardiac output or decreased systemic vascular resistance.
- Tachycardia: The heart rate increases, compensating for the decreased cardiac output, helping maintain blood pressure and perfusion.
- Myocardial dysfunction: In some types of shock, for example, cardiogenic shock, there may be impaired myocardial contractility, leading to reduced stroke volume and cardiac output.

Fluid shifts: In some cases, shock can cause fluid to shift from the intravascular space (blood vessels) into the interstitial spaces, leading to oedema and worsening hypovolaemia.

Endothelial dysfunction: Shock can impair the function of the endothelium (the inner lining of blood vessels). This can result in increased vascular permeability, leading to leakage of fluid and proteins into the interstitial spaces, further exacerbating oedema.

Coagulation and microthrombi: In response to shock, the body may activate the coagulation cascade and form microthrombi (small blood clots) within the microcirculation. This can impair blood flow to vital organs and contribute to organ dysfunction.

Organ dysfunction and failure: Prolonged or severe shock can lead to dysfunction and failure of multiple organ systems, including the heart, lungs, kidneys, liver and central nervous system. This can manifest as acute respiratory distress syndrome (ARDS), acute kidney injury (AKI), hepatic dysfunction, altered mental status and more.

Systemic inflammation: Shock can trigger a systemic inflammatory response, often referred to as systemic inflammatory response syndrome (SIRS) or sepsis if infection is present. This further exacerbates organ dysfunction and can lead to a cascade of immune responses.

Multiple organ dysfunction syndrome (MODS): In severe and prolonged shock, the dysfunction of multiple organ systems can progress to MODS, where two or more organs fail. MODS is a life-threatening condition with a high mortality rate.

Understanding these pathophysiological changes associated with shock is crucial for healthcare professionals, as early recognition and intervention are essential for improving outcomes in those experiencing shock. Treatment strategies aim to restore adequate tissue perfusion, address the underlying cause(s) and support organ function.

SHOCK: SIGNS AND SYMPTOMS

There are a range of signs and symptoms people may present with in relation to shock; Jones (2023) and Migliozzi (2021) discuss these further. There may be altered mental status, this is a common sign of shock, including lethargy, confusion and drowsiness. The person's hands and feet may be pale, cool, clammy and often cyanotic, as are the earlobes, nose and nailbeds. If the patient has a darker complexion, check the inner eyelids and mucous membranes for a loss of colour.

Capillary filling time is prolonged, and, except in distributive shock, the skin appears greyish or dusky and moist. Obvious diaphoresis may occur. Peripheral pulses are weak and typically rapid; often, only a femoral or carotid pulse is palpable. Tachypnoea and hyperventilation may be present. Blood pressure tends to be low or unobtainable. Urine output is low.

Distributive shock will cause similar symptoms; however, the skin may appear warm or flushed, particularly during sepsis. The pulse may be bounding as opposed to weak. In septic shock, pyrexia, possibly preceded by chills, is usually present. Some patients with anaphylactic shock have urticaria or wheezing.

Other symptoms such as chest pain, dyspnoea and abdominal pain may be due to the underlying disease or secondary organ failure.

PATHOPHYSIOLOGICAL CHANGES ASSOCIATED WITH CARDIOGENIC SHOCK

The pathophysiology of cardiogenic shock is poorly understood due to a paucity of high-quality clinical data (Hill 2023). Cardiogenic shock is a complex condition that is rooted in primary cardiac dysfunction, which results in reduced cardiac output and inadequate tissue perfusion; it is a severe form of heart failure (Menzies-Gow 2019). The body's compensatory responses initially aim to maintain vital organ perfusion but can ultimately exacerbate the condition, leading to a vicious cycle of deteriorating cardiac function. Effective management of cardiogenic shock requires addressing both the underlying cardiac problem and supporting organ function to improve patient outcomes.

Lear and Thompson (2019) note that cardiogenic shock results in a low cardiac output state leading to life-threatening end-organ perfusion. It is caused by disorders that impair the function of the heart. Acute myocardial infarction with left ventricular dysfunction is the most common cause of cardiogenic shock. The damage that occurs to the myocardium prevents the heart from pumping effectively; this results in a fall in cardiac output as well as blood pressure with tissue hypoperfusion. Paradoxically, the compensatory mechanisms that would usually function to maintain end-organ perfusion are actually pathological in the case

Table 5.3 Mechanisms associated with cardiogenic shock

Mechanism	Cause
Impaired myocardial contractility	• Myocardial ischaemia
	• Myocardial infarction
	• Myocarditis
	• Drugs
Abnormalities of cardiac rhythm	• Tachycardia
	• Bradycardia
Cardiac structural disorder	• Acute mitral valve regurgitation
	• Acute aortic regurgitation
	• Ruptured intraventricular septum
	• Prosthetic valve malfunction

Source: Adapted from Hill (2023); Hagler et al. (2023).

of cardiogenic shock (Lear and Thompson 2019). The catecholamines that are released produce tachycardia, vasoconstriction and increased cardiac contractility. These compensatory responses will increase myocardial oxygen demand and the workload of the left ventricle. This can potentially cause extension of the infarct and result in further compromise of left ventricular function. As afterload increases due to peripheral vasoconstriction and increased systemic vascular resistance, the left ventricle cannot empty effectively. As a result, pressure rises in the left atrium, the pulmonary circulation, and the right side of the heart. Pulmonary oedema ensues and gaseous exchange in the alveoli is impeded due to the presence of fluid in the lungs and the problem of tissue hypoxia, in the context of shock, is exacerbated. See Table 5.3 for the mechanisms associated with cardiogenic shock.

EPIDEMIOLOGY

Mortality in cardiogenic shock remains high (Ordonez and Garan 2022). Nearly 1 in 10 patients suffering from a heart attack will develop cardiogenic shock and up to half of patients will not survive to hospital discharge. Such high death rates are attributable in a number of ways to delays in recognition of cardiogenic shock and ensuring timely access to the evidence-based interventions and expertise that is required for positive patient outcomes (Intensive Care Society 2022).

As well as uncertainty about the accurate prevalence of cardiogenic shock, there is a paucity of data that illustrates how care is delivered for people with cardiogenic shock. As data is scarce, it can be tentatively suggested that there will be significant variation in care, as well as equity of access.

Currently, there is a lack of epidemiological data regarding cardiogenic shock (Intensive Care Society 2022). Epidemiological data is invaluable for understanding the scope, impact and underlying factors of cardiogenic shock. It informs clinical practices, research and public health efforts, ultimately contributing to improved patient outcomes and the prevention of this life-threatening condition.

RISK FACTORS

It is essential to recognise and manage the risk factors and underlying conditions to reduce the risk of cardiogenic shock. Prompt medical attention and appropriate treatment are crucial in managing this life-threatening condition. Table 5.4 provides an overview of risk factors that are associated with cardiogenic shock.

Table 5.4 Risk factors associated with cardiogenic shock

Risk factor	Discussion
Myocardial infarction	The most common cause of cardiogenic shock is myocardial infarction that damages a significant portion of the heart muscle, reducing its ability to contract effectively.
Severe heart failure	Individuals with advanced heart failure may be at a higher risk of developing cardiogenic shock. Heart failure can be caused by various underlying conditions, including coronary artery disease, cardiomyopathy and valvular heart disease.
Cardiomyopathy	Certain types of cardiomyopathy, such as dilated cardiomyopathy and hypertrophic cardiomyopathy, can weaken the heart muscle and increase the risk of cardiogenic shock.
Valvular heart disease	Conditions such as severe aortic stenosis or mitral regurgitation can put additional strain on the heart and lead to cardiogenic shock if left untreated.
Arrhythmias	Severe arrhythmias, especially ventricular tachycardia or fibrillation, can disrupt the heart's normal rhythm and cause cardiogenic shock.
Cardiac arrest	A sudden cardiac arrest, where the heart stops beating, can lead to cardiogenic shock if not promptly treated with cardiopulmonary resuscitation and defibrillation.
Cardiac surgery	Certain cardiac surgical procedures, such as coronary artery bypass grafting or valve replacement, can be associated with a risk of cardiogenic shock, although this risk is generally low.
Drug-related causes	Some medications or substances, such as certain toxins, can have a toxic effect on the heart and increase the risk of cardiogenic shock.
Prior coronary artery disease	A history of heart attacks or coronary artery disease can increase the likelihood of subsequent cardiac events, including cardiogenic shock.
Age and gender	Older individuals, particularly men, are at a higher risk of developing cardiogenic shock, although it can affect people of all ages and genders.
Diabetes	Individuals with poorly controlled diabetes may have an increased risk of cardiovascular complications, including cardiogenic shock.
Hypertension	Uncontrolled high blood pressure can lead to heart muscle damage and increase the risk of cardiogenic shock.
Overweight and obesity	Overweight and obesity are risk factors for cardiogenic shock primarily because they contribute to the development of other cardiovascular conditions, such as coronary artery disease and heart failure, which are leading causes of cardiogenic shock.

Source: Adapted from National Heart, Lung, and Blood Institute (2022).

CLINICAL PRESENTATION

The clinical presentation related to cardiogenic shock occurs as a reaction to the loss of oxygen-rich blood in the body. The symptoms a person may experience depend on how quickly the blood pressure drops and how low it gets. Some individuals may experience mild symptoms initially; however, others may have no symptoms and then immediately lose consciousness. Hill (2023) notes the following as red flag symptoms of cardiogenic shock:

- Sudden drop in blood pressure
- Bradycardia
- Raised jugular venous pressure
- Swollen ankles (oedema)
- Pale, blue hue to white skin tones and chalky pale discolouration to dark skin tones
- Cold hands and feet
- Sweaty skin
- Confusion
- Decreased consciousness
- Tachypnoea
- Cardiac arrest

CLINICAL INVESTIGATIONS AND DIAGNOSIS

A medical history is taken and a physical examination performed. The investigations required for a patient with cardiogenic shock are based upon the extent of damage to the heart and the effect this has on the major organs (Dutton and Elliot 2021). The following are performed when examining the patient:

- Examine hands and feet: To determine the temperature and presence of oedema.
- Palpate pulse: Assess rate and rhythm.
- Auscultate heart and lungs: Listen for unusual sounds or heart rhythms.
- Measure and monitor urine output: Provides valuable information about haemodynamic status and kidney function.
- Measure and monitor blood pressure: Aids in diagnosis and classification of the condition, guides treatment decisions, monitors response to therapy, assesses risk of complications and helps assess organ perfusion.

POTENTIAL INVESTIGATIONS

- Chest X-ray: Assesses structures in and around the chest.
- Coronary angiography: Uses a contrast dye and X-ray images to detect blockages in coronary arteries caused by plaque buildup.

- Echocardiography: Also known as echo, uses sound waves to create moving images of the heart showing size and shape and how well the heart is pumping blood. Doppler ultrasound shows how well blood flows through the chambers of the heart and valves.
- Electrocardiogram (ECG): Detects and records the heart's electrical activity, how fast the heart is beating and cardiac rhythm.

Other tests include arterial blood gas analysis and other blood tests to assess how well the heart, liver and kidneys are working and to determine increased lactate or lactic acid levels.

MANAGEMENT

Patients with cardiogenic shock require defined pathways of escalation and care with the intention of improving survival; cardiogenic shock is treatable if diagnosed and treated quickly. Patients should be included in all decision-making processes and fully informed of any proposed interventions with an opportunity to agree to or to decline treatment. Care provision should be respectful of, and responsive to, individual preferences, needs and values, ensuring that the patient's values guide all clinical decisions (Intensive Care Society 2022).

Treatment focuses on getting blood flowing effectively and protecting organs from damage. For some people, they may need a heart transplant or a permanently implanted device (ventricular assist devices) to help keep blood flowing to the heart. If not treated quickly, cardiogenic shock can be fatal or lead to organ failure or brain injury. Possible management options are identified in Table 5.5.

In Figure 5.2, potential patient outcomes for people presenting with cardiogenic shock are described.

HEALTH TEACHING

Health promotion for a person who has experienced cardiogenic shock is essential to reduce the risk of future cardiac events, improve overall health and enhance quality of life. After surviving cardiogenic shock, individuals should work closely with healthcare providers,

Table 5.5 Potential management options

Medication	Medical procedures	Surgery
- Analgesia - Aspirin - Platelet glycoprotein IIb/IIIa receptor blockers - Anticoagulants - Vasopressor/inotropic agents	- Angioplasty and stenting - Revascularisation - Intra-aortic balloon pump counterpulsation	- Coronary artery bypass surgery - Surgery to repair an injury to the heart (i.e. a tear in the heart, valve replacement) - Ventricular assist devices (heart pumps) - Heart transplant

Health Teaching 91

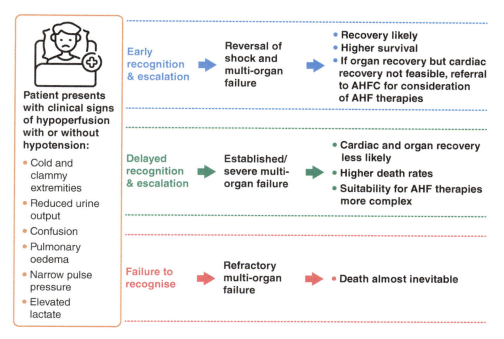

FIGURE 5.2 Patient outcomes for people presenting with cardiogenic shock and the importance of early recognition. AHF: advanced heart failure; AHFC: advanced heart failure centre. *Source:* Intensive Care Society (2022).

developing a comprehensive plan addressing specific needs and risk factors. These are some key aspects of health promotion:

- Participation in a cardiac rehabilitation programme is highly recommended.
- Compliance with prescribed medications is essential for managing underlying heart conditions and preventing future cardiac events.
- Adopting a heart-healthy diet can significantly reduce the risk of future heart problems. Usually involves reducing saturated fats, cholesterol, sodium and processed foods while increasing fruits, vegetables, whole grains and lean proteins.
- Regular physical activity is essential for cardiovascular health. An appropriate exercise plan tailored to the individual's abilities and medical condition is advocated.
- Quitting smoking is one of the most important steps to improve heart health.
- Achieving and maintaining a healthy weight can reduce the strain on the heart.
- Chronic stress has the potential to negatively impact heart health. Learning stress management techniques such as meditation, yoga or mindfulness can be beneficial.
- Ongoing monitoring and follow-up appointments are essential to assess cardiac function, adjust medications and address any emerging issues.
- Keeping blood pressure within a healthy range is crucial.

- If the person has diabetes, management of blood glucose levels is essential.
- Individuals should be informed about the signs and symptoms of heart-related issues and encouraged to seek prompt medical attention if they experience chest pain, shortness of breath or other concerning symptoms.
- Building a strong support system, including family, friends and healthcare providers, can help the individual manage their health effectively and cope with any emotional challenges that may arise.
- Addressing mental health and emotional well-being is vital. Experiencing a life-threatening event such as cardiogenic shock can lead to anxiety, depression or post-traumatic stress.
- Routine screenings for heart disease risk factors, such as cholesterol levels, blood pressure and blood glucose are important for early detection and prevention.

Health promotion for those who have survived cardiogenic shock is a lifelong commitment to maintaining heart health. A personalised and multidisciplinary approach, involving healthcare providers, nutritionists, physical therapists and mental health professionals, can help individuals make sustainable lifestyle changes and reduce the risk of future cardiac events.

CONCLUSION

Cardiogenic shock is a critical condition that requires prompt recognition and intervention. Understanding the nuances of cardiogenic shock is crucial, as it is a life-threatening state that can be encountered in various settings (clinical and out of settings).

Cardiogenic shock demands swift recognition and appropriate intervention. Those who provide care and support to people should familiarise themselves with the causes, clinical presentation, assessment and interventions for cardiogenic shock to provide safe and effective care to patients. A collaborative approach, involving teamwork and communication among healthcare professionals, is essential for the successful management of cardiogenic shock.

GLOSSARY OF TERMS

Afterload: The resistance against which the heart must pump blood, often increased in cardiogenic shock.

Bradycardia: An abnormally slow heart rate may be seen in cardiogenic shock.

Cardiac output: The amount of blood the heart pumps per minute, an important factor in maintaining adequate tissue perfusion.

Cardiogenic shock: A life-threatening condition where the heart fails to pump blood effectively, leading to inadequate oxygen and nutrient supply to vital organs.

Electrocardiogram: A test recording electrical activity of the heart, often used to diagnose myocardial infarction.

Hypotension: Abnormally low blood pressure, a common symptom of cardiogenic shock.

Hypoxaemia: Insufficient oxygen levels in the blood, often seen in shock due to impaired tissue oxygenation.

Lactic acidosis: An increase in lactic acid levels in the blood due to tissue hypoxia, a common finding in shock.

Myocardial infarction: A heart attack occurs when there is a sudden blockage of blood flow to a part of heart muscle, often leading to cardiogenic shock.

Preload: Volume of blood in the heart's ventricles at the end of diastole, which influences the heart's stroke volume.

Pulmonary oedema: Accumulation of fluid in the lungs due to increased pressure in the pulmonary circulation, a common complication of cardiogenic shock.

Shock: A critical medical condition characterised by inadequate tissue perfusion, resulting in organ dysfunction and potential failure.

Stroke volume: The amount of blood ejected from the heart with each beat.

Tissue perfusion: The delivery of oxygen and nutrients to cells and removal of waste products, a critical aspect of shock management.

Troponin: A cardiac biomarker that becomes elevated in the blood after a myocardial infarction or heart muscle damage.

MULTIPLE CHOICE QUESTION

1. What is the primary cause of cardiogenic shock?
   a) Hypovolemia
   b) Cardiac tamponade
   c) Myocardial infarction
   d) Pulmonary embolism

2. Which of the following is NOT a common symptom of cardiogenic shock?
   a) Hypotension
   b) Tachycardia
   c) Hypothermia
   d) Shortness of breath

3. Which cardiac biomarker is typically elevated in cardiogenic shock due to myocardial infarction?
   a) Creatinine
   b) Troponin
   c) Bilirubin
   d) Haemoglobin

4. What is the most common cause of cardiogenic shock in the elderly population?
   a) Pulmonary embolism
   b) Aortic dissection
   c) Acute myocardial infarction
   d) Cardiac tamponade

5. Cardiogenic shock can lead to what type of organ dysfunction?
   a) Renal failure
   b) Neurological impairment
   c) Gastrointestinal bleeding
   d) All of the above

6. Which diagnostic imaging test can help identify the underlying cause of cardiogenic shock?
   a) Electrocardiogram (ECG)
   b) Chest X-ray
   c) Magnetic resonance imaging (MRI)
   d) Lumbar puncture

7. Which intervention is a priority when caring for a patient with cardiogenic shock?
   a) Administering oral medications
   b) Monitoring urine output
   c) Applying cold compresses to the extremities
   d) Promoting physical activity

8. Cardiogenic shock can lead to pulmonary oedema due to:
   a) Decreased intrathoracic pressure
   b) Increased left ventricular pressure
   c) Increased alveolar ventilation
   d) Decreased capillary permeability

9. Which of the following clinical findings is an early sign of cardiogenic shock?
   a) Bradycardia
   b) Hypertension
   c) Cool, clammy skin
   d) Hyperthermia

10. Which of the following factors may exacerbate cardiogenic shock?
    a) Hyperventilation
    b) Fluid overload
    c) High-dose aspirin
    d) Non-rebreather mask

REFERENCES

British Medical Journal Best Practice (2022). *Cardiac Arrest*. London: BMJ Publishing Group [Free Full-text]. https://bestpractice.bmj.com.

Chadick, A. (2021). Basic first aid (Chapter 18). In: *The Nursing Associate's Handbook of Clinical Skills* (ed. I. Peate). Oxford: Wiley.

Dutton, H. and Elliot, S. (2021). The person with acute cardiovascular problems (Chapter 6). In: *Acute Nursing Care*, 2e (eds. I. Peate and H. Dutton). London: Routledge.

Hagler, D., Harding, M.M., Kwong, J. et al. (2023). *Lewis's Medical-Surgical Nursing*, 12e. St Louis: Elsevier.

Hill, B. (2023). Shock (Chapter 8). In: *Fundamentals of Critical Care* (eds. I. Peate and B. Hill). Oxford: Wiley.

Intensive Care Society (2022). Shock to survival. https://ics.ac.uk/resource/shock-to-survival-report.html (accessed October 2023).

Jones, N.P. (2023). The principles of fluid and electrolyte imbalance and shock (Chapter 25). In: *Nursing Practice*, 3e (eds. I. Peate and A. Mitchell). Oxford: Wiley.

Lear, R. and Thompson, S. (2019). Recognising and manging shock (Chapter 18). In: *Alexander's Nursing Practice*, 5e (ed. I. Peate). London: Elsevier.

Menzies-Gow, E. (2019). Nursing patients with cardiovascular disorders (Chapter 3). In: *Alexander's Nursing Practice,* 5e (ed. I. Peate). London: Elsevier.

Migliozzi, J.G. (2021). Shock (Chapter 6). In: *Fundamentals of Applied Pathophysiology,* 4e (ed. I. Peate). Oxford: Wiley.

National Heart, Lung and Blood Institute (2022). Cardiogenic shock. Causes and risk factors. https://www.nhlbi.nih.gov/health/cardiogenic-shock/causes (accessed October 2023).

Ordonez, C. and Garan, A.R. (2022). The landscape of cardiogenic shock: epidemiology and current definitions. *Current Opinion Cardiology* 37 (3): 236–240. doi:10.1097/HCO.0000000000000957.

Perkins, G.D., Nolan, J.P., Soar, J. et al. (2021a). Epidemiology of cardiac arrest guidelines. https://www.resus.org.uk/library/2021-resuscitation-guidelines/epidemiology-cardiac-arrest-guidelines (accessed October 2023).

Perkins, G.D., Colquhoun, M., Deakin, C.D. et al. (2021b). Adult basic life support guidelines. https://www.resus.org.uk/library/2021-resuscitation-guidelines/adult-basic-life-support-guidelines (accessed October 2023).

Tsao, C.W., Aday, A.W., Almarzooq, Z.I. et al. (2023). Heart disease and stroke statistics-2023 update: a report from the American Heart Association. *Circulation* 147 (8): e622. doi:10.1161/CIR.0000000000001123.

CHAPTER 6 Angina

Angina, also known as angina pectoris, is pain (or constricting discomfort) in the chest, neck, shoulders, jaw or arms caused by an insufficient blood supply to the myocardium (National Institute for Health and Care Excellence [NICE] 2016). It is a common symptom of coronary heart disease. Angina is a complex clinical scenario that is characterised by different pathophysiological mechanisms; frequently it is caused by microvascular abnormalities (see Sardella and Mancone 2018).

The word 'angina' is derived from the Latin word 'angere', which means 'to strangle' or 'to choke'. In medical terminology, 'angina' had originally referred to any condition or symptom that caused a sensation of choking or suffocation. Over time, angina became specifically associated with chest pain or discomfort. It is now referred to as 'angina pectoris', pectoris is also Latin and means 'of the chest' or 'pertaining to the chest.'

Usually, angina is caused by coronary artery disease, atherosclerotic plaques located in the coronary arteries that cause a progressive narrowing of the lumen, along with symptoms that occur when blood flow does not provide adequate amounts of oxygen to the myocardium at times when oxygen demand increases. Angina can also be caused by valvular disease (for example, aortic stenosis), hypertrophic obstructive cardiomyopathy or hypertensive heart disease, but this is less common (NICE 2016).

Stable angina usually occurs predictably with physical exertion or emotional stress, lasts for no more than 10 minutes (usually less) and is relieved within minutes of rest, as well as sublingual nitrates.

Unstable angina is new onset angina or abrupt deterioration in previously stable angina; this often occurs at rest. Unstable angina will often require immediate admission or referral to the hospital.

Usually, angina is caused by coronary artery disease. Atherosclerotic plaques in the coronary arteries cause progressive narrowing of the lumen and symptoms occur when blood flow does not provide adequate amounts of oxygen to the myocardium at times when oxygen demand increases (for example, when exercising).

STABLE ANGINA

Stable angina is a type of angina pectoris, a medical condition that is characterised by chest pain or discomfort. Stable angina, however, has specific characteristics that distinguish it from other types of angina and heart-related chest pain. Here are some key features of chronic stable angina:

Predictable episodes: Stable angina is characterised by chest pain or discomfort that occurs predictably and transiently during certain activities or under specific conditions. These triggering factors increase the heart's demand for oxygen, and the chest pain arises because the heart muscle does not receive enough oxygen-rich blood during these times (Ashelford and Taylor 2023).

Relief with rest or medication: The chest pain or discomfort in stable angina usually subsides with rest or the use of medications such as GTN, a vasodilator that dilates the coronary arteries and improves blood flow to the heart muscle.

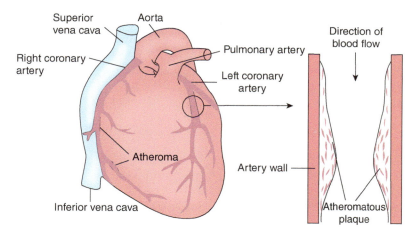

FIGURE 6.1   Blockage of the coronary artery

Consistency of symptoms: The pattern and severity of symptoms in stable angina tend to remain relatively consistent over time. The individual often knows what activities or situations can trigger their chest pain.

No or minimal symptoms at rest: Unlike unstable angina, where chest pain can occur at rest and is often a sign of a more serious issue, stable angina typically does not manifest at rest. It is brought on by specific triggers.

Caused by coronary artery disease: Stable angina is most commonly associated with coronary artery disease, where the coronary arteries that supply blood to the heart muscle become narrowed or blocked by atherosclerotic plaques (see Figure 6.1). The narrowing of these arteries restricts blood flow and oxygen delivery to the heart muscle.

SILENT ANGINA

Also known as silent ischaemia angina refers to a condition in which a person experiences a lack of blood flow and oxygen to the heart muscle (ischaemia) without feeling the typical symptoms of angina, such as chest pain or discomfort. This lack of symptoms makes it 'silent' because the individual is often unaware that they are experiencing a heart-related issue. Silent angina is a concerning condition because it can go unnoticed and untreated, potentially leading to serious heart problems. Menzies-Gow (2019) suggests that the event is not entirely silent, as patients often experience associated symptoms, for example, shortness of breath, fatigue, nausea and vomiting or severe distress. Silent angina can occur in various situations, including:

During exercise: Some individuals may have ischaemia during physical activity or stress testing, but they do not experience chest pain or discomfort. This is often discovered when an electrocardiogram (ECG) or other diagnostic tests show signs of ischaemia (Ashelford and Taylor 2023).

During sleep: Silent angina can also occur during sleep or periods of rest when the heart's oxygen demand is lower. These episodes may be detected through monitoring devices that record heart activity while the person is asleep.

In people with diabetes: People with diabetes are at an increased risk of silent angina because diabetes can affect the nerves that transmit pain signals. As a result, they may not feel chest pain even when they have reduced blood flow to the heart.

In older adults: Older individuals may have diminished sensitivity to pain or may attribute their symptoms to other causes, making it more likely for them to be aware they are experiencing silent angina.

PRINZMETAL'S ANGINA

This type of angina is also known as variant angina or vasospastic angina. It is a relatively rare form of angina pectoris, a condition characterised by chest pain or discomfort due to reduced blood flow to the heart muscle. Prinzmetal's angina is distinct from the more common form of angina stable angina, as it has unique characteristics, which include:

Vasospasm: Prinzmetal's angina is primarily caused by the sudden and temporary narrowing (spasm) of the coronary arteries that supply blood to the heart. This spasm reduces blood flow and oxygen delivery to the heart muscle, resulting in chest pain or discomfort (Hagler et al. 2023).

Triggers: Unlike stable angina, Prinzmetal's angina frequently occurs at rest, during sleep or with minimal physical activity. Certain triggers, such as exposure to cold temperatures or emotional stress, can provoke these spasms.

Cyclic patterns: Prinzmetal's angina often follows a cyclic pattern, with episodes of chest pain occurring at predictable times. These episodes can be frequent or sporadic.

Response to medications: Glyceryl trinitrate (GTN), a medication that dilates coronary arteries and improves blood flow, is often effective in relieving chest pain associated with Prinzmetal's angina.

ECG changes: During an episode of Prinzmetal's angina, ECG recordings may show specific changes, for example, ST-segment elevation, which can help diagnose the condition.

MICROVASCULAR ANGINA

Microvascular angina, also known as cardiac syndrome X, is a type of angina pectoris. Microvascular angina, however, differs from typical angina in several ways:

Affected blood vessels: In microvascular angina, chest pain occurs due to dysfunction or abnormalities in the tiny blood vessels (microvessels) that branch off from the main coronary arteries and supply blood to the heart muscle. These microvessels are too small to be seen on standard coronary angiograms, and this is why this condition is often referred to as 'microvascular'.

Normal coronary arteries: Unlike traditional angina, where chest pain is typically associated with blockages or narrowing of the large coronary arteries (coronary artery disease), those with microvascular angina often have angiographically normal coronary arteries. The main coronary arteries appear normal on imaging tests, making a diagnosis a challenge.

Triggers and characteristics: The chest pain or discomfort in microvascular angina can be triggered by physical exertion, emotional stress or other factors that increase the heart's oxygen demand, similar to stable angina. The pain may have characteristics similar to other types of angina, for example, a squeezing or pressure-like sensation in the chest.

Potential causes: The exact cause of microvascular angina is not fully understood; however, it is believed to involve dysfunction of the microvessels that limit blood flow to the heart muscle (British Heart Foundation 2017a). Factors such as endothelial dysfunction (these are abnormalities in the lining of the blood vessels), inflammation and abnormalities in the microvascular structure may play a role.

PATHOPHYSIOLOGICAL CHANGES ASSOCIATED WITH ANGINA

Angina pectoris is a clinical syndrome of precordial discomfort or pressure due to transient myocardial ischaemia without infarction. It is typically brought on by exertion or psychological stress; angina is relieved by rest or sublingual nitroglycerine (GTN).

Table 6.1 differentiates between angina and myocardial infarction (see also Chapter 3 of this book).

In summary, angina is a symptom of reduced blood flow to the heart muscle as a result of narrowed coronary arteries: it is usually temporary and manageable. Myocardial infarction, however, is a more severe condition that is caused by a complete blockage of a coronary artery. This leads to the death of heart muscle tissue and requires immediate medical intervention. Both conditions are related to heart health and they should be evaluated and treated by healthcare professionals. Figure 6.2 depicts a healthy heart, angina pectoris and myocardial infarction.

Table 6.1 Angina and myocardial infarction

	Angina	Myocardial infarction
Cause	Angina is typically caused by a temporary reduction in blood flow to the heart muscle (myocardium) as a result of narrowed or blocked coronary arteries. It can often occur during physical exertion or at times of stress when the heart's demand for oxygen increases and the narrowed arteries are unable to supply enough blood to meet this demand.	Myocardial infarction occurs when there is a prolonged and severe reduction or complete blockage of blood flow to a part of the heart muscle. This is usually due to the complete blockage of a coronary artery, often caused by the rupture of an atherosclerotic plaque and the subsequent blood clot formation.
Pain and duration	The chest pain or discomfort in angina is usually temporary (1–3 minutes, can be up to 20 minutes) and this will subside with rest or medication. It is often described by patients as a feeling of pressure, tightness or discomfort in the chest, and it may radiate to other areas such as the arms, neck, jaw, shoulder or back.	In myocardial infarction, the chest pain is typically more severe and prolonged than angina (20 minutes to several hours) and it does not improve with rest or medication. It is often described as crushing and intense, and it may be associated with other symptoms such as shortness of breath, nausea, vomiting, cold sweats and anxiety.
Damage to heart muscle	Angina does not typically cause permanent damage to the heart muscle since it is a result of temporary oxygen deprivation.	Myocardial infarction involves the death of a portion of the heart muscle due to a prolonged lack of blood flow. This has the potential to lead to permanent damage and potentially life-threatening complications if not treated promptly.

(Continued)

Table 6.1 *(Continued)*

	Angina	Myocardial infarction
Treatment and urgency	Treatment for angina involves managing the symptoms and addressing the underlying cause, such as coronary artery disease. Medications, lifestyle changes and procedures such as angioplasty or stent placement may be used.	Myocardial infarction is a medical emergency and requires immediate treatment; this is crucial. This typically involves restoring blood flow to the blocked coronary artery as quickly as possible, often through procedures such as angioplasty and stent placement or thrombolytic therapy. Medications to reduce the heart's workload and prevent further complications are also administered.
Factors that may aggravate	Frequent exertion, particularly in the cold; meals; emotional stress. Can occur at rest.	Not always triggered by exertion.
Associated symptoms	There may be dyspnoea, nausea and diaphoresis.	Dyspnoea, nausea, vomiting, diaphoresis, fatigue and weakness.

Source: Bickley et al. (2023). With permission of Wolters Kluwer Health, Inc.

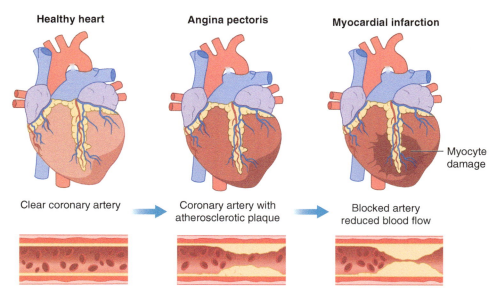

FIGURE 6.2 Coronary artery disease depicting a healthy heart, angina pectoris and myocardial infarction

Angina may be stable or unstable. In stable angina, the relationship between workload or demand and ischaemia is usually relatively predictable. Unstable angina is clinically worsening angina, that is to say, angina at rest or with increasing frequency and/or intensity of episodes.

Atherosclerotic arterial narrowing is not totally fixed; it varies with the normal fluctuations in arterial tone occurring in everyone. Therefore, more people have angina in the morning, when arterial tone is relatively high. Furthermore, abnormal endothelial function may contribute to variations in arterial tone.

As the myocardium becomes ischaemic, coronary sinus blood pH falls, cellular potassium is lost, lactate accumulates, ECG abnormalities appear and ventricular function (systolic and diastolic) deteriorates. Left ventricular diastolic pressure usually increases during angina, sometimes inducing pulmonary congestion and dyspnoea. The exact mechanism by which ischaemia causes discomfort is unclear; it may involve nerve stimulation by hypoxic metabolites.

EPIDEMIOLOGY

Angina pectoris is a common clinical manifestation of ischaemic heart disease with an estimated prevalence of 3–4% in UK adults. Ford and Berry (2020) inform that annually, there are over 250 000 invasive coronary angiograms carried out, with over 20 000 new cases of angina. The healthcare resource use is substantial with over 110 000 inpatient episodes annually that lead to substantial associated morbidity.

RISK FACTORS

There may be a higher risk of angina because of age, sex, race, medical conditions, family history and genetics, environment, occupation or lifestyle. Understanding risk factors can help diagnose the condition and prepare a treatment plan that is tailor-made in response to individual needs.

AGE

Genetic or lifestyle factors may cause plaque to build up in the arteries as the person ages. The risk of coronary heart disease and angina increases as a person ages.

Those who have vasospastic angina (also known as Prinzmetal's angina or variant angina) are often younger than those who have more common types of angina.

ENVIRONMENT OR OCCUPATION

Angina may be linked to air pollution. Particle pollution can include dust from roads, farms, dry riverbeds, construction sites and mines.

A person's occupation can increase the risk of angina, for example, work that limits a person's available time for sleep, work that involves high stress, requires long periods of sitting or standing, is noisy or exposes the employee to potential hazards such as radiation.

FAMILY HISTORY AND GENETICS

Coronary heart disease often runs in families and people who have no lifestyle-related risk factors can develop heart disease. These factors suggest that genes are involved in coronary heart disease and can affect a person's risk of developing angina.

LIFESTYLE HABITS

The more heart disease risk factors a person has, the greater they are at risk of developing angina. The main lifestyle risk factors for angina include:

- Alcohol use, for vasospastic angina.
- Illegal drug use, which can cause the heart to race or damage blood vessels.
- Lack of physical activity.
- Smoking tobacco or long-term exposure to second-hand smoke.
- Stress.
- Unhealthy eating patterns.

OTHER MEDICAL CONDITIONS

In some medical conditions, the heart needs more oxygen-rich blood than the body can supply, raising the risk of angina. They include:

- Anaemia
- Cardiomyopathy
- Heart conditions, such as heart failure, heart valve diseases or high blood pressure
- Inflammation
- Metabolic syndrome

MEDICAL PROCEDURES

Heart procedures, for example, stent placement, percutaneous coronary intervention (PCI), or coronary artery bypass grafting (CABG) may trigger coronary spasms and angina. Sometimes, non-cardiac surgery can also trigger unstable angina or vasospastic angina.

ETHNICITY

Some groups of people are at higher risk of developing coronary heart disease and one of its main symptoms, angina. Studies in the UK consistently show a higher incidence, prevalence and mortality from cardiovascular disease in South Asian groups compared with the White group or national average. South Asian groups have the highest mortality from heart disease and also develop heart disease at a younger age (Raleigh 2023).

GENDER

Angina affects men and women. In men, the chance of having heart disease starts to rise at the age of 45 years. Before 55 years, women have a lower risk of heart disease than men. After 55, the risk rises in women and men. Women who have already had a heart attack have a higher chance of developing angina compared with men. Microvascular angina most often begins in women around the time of menopause.

Table 6.2 PQRST assessment of angina

P	Precipitating events	What events or activities precipitated the pain or discomfort, for example, stressful event, exercise or resting?
Q	Quality of pain	What does the pain or discomfort feel like, does it feel like pressure, dull, tight, squeezing, aching or heaviness?
R	Region (location) and radiation of pain	Are you able to point to where the pain or discomfort is located? Does the pain or discomfort radiate to other places such as the neck, arms, jaw, back, elbow or shoulder?
S	Severity of pain	On a scale, where 0 equals no pain or discomfort and 10 refers to the most severe pain or discomfort imaginable, what number would you score your pain or discomfort?
T	Timing	When did the pain or discomfort come on? Has it changed since then? Have you experienced pain or discomfort like this before?

CLINICAL PRESENTATION

It is important to note that the clinical presentation of angina may vary from person to person, some individuals may have atypical or subtle symptoms. Angina can be a sign of significant heart disease and prompt evaluation is essential for appropriate diagnosis and management. Clinical presentations for the various types of angina have already been discussed. Chest pain or discomfort are hallmark symptoms of angina. See Table 6.2 for PQRST assessment of angina.

CLINICAL INVESTIGATIONS AND DIAGNOSIS

People with stable angina should have the diagnosis made after a carefully obtained patient history and clinical assessment have been undertaken. Diagnosis of stable angina can often be made by taking a patient history (Clare 2019). According to the Scottish Intercollegiate Guidelines Network (SIGN 2018), clinical history is the key component in the evaluation of a patient with angina; the diagnosis can often be made based on clinical history alone.

Diagnosis is by history, symptoms, ECG and myocardial imaging. Blood tests will also be required and an exercise stress test is undertaken, to determine how well the heart is working. As part of a physical examination, blood pressure is measured and the pulse rate, rhythm and depth are recorded and the temperature is taken. The chest, lungs and abdomen are auscultated, palpated and percussed. See Table 6.3.

Various scoring systems are available to assist in the assessment of patients with chest pain and stable angina. An accurate clinical assessment is of the greatest importance. There are a number of typical characteristics, which should increase the likelihood of making a diagnosis of angina. Including, for example:

- Type of discomfort, this is often described as tight, constricting, dull or heavy.
- Location, often retrosternal or left side of chest and can radiate to left arm, neck, jaw and back.
- Relation to exertion, angina is often brought on by exertion or emotional stress and eased with rest.
- Duration, typically the symptoms last up to several minutes after exertion or emotional stress has stopped.
- Other factors, angina may be precipitated by cold weather or after a large meal.

Table 6.3 Tests and investigations

Test/procedure	Discussion
Electrocardiogram (ECG)	Can help to recognise types of angina and other serious heart problems. Some ECG tracings can be a sign of unstable angina or vasospastic angina. However, the ECG may sometimes be normal, even if the person has angina.
Chest X-ray	Useful for screening for lung disorders and other causes of chest pain, such as pneumonia and heart failure. A chest X-ray alone is not enough to diagnose angina or coronary heart disease, it can help rule out other causes of symptoms.
Blood tests	Can measure the level of cardiac troponin in the blood to help determine unstable angina from myocardial infarction. Other blood tests check levels of other proteins, certain fats, cholesterol and glucose in the blood.
Echocardiogram	Also called echo, can show how well the heart pumps blood to the rest of the body. May help identify problems inside the heart, for example, blood clots or damaged heart valves.
Cardiac magnetic resonance imaging	Along with other non-invasive tests, it can help check for problems with the heart's movement or blood supply.
Stress testing	This test assesses how well the heart works during exercise. A stress test can help confirm whether coronary heart disease is causing angina symptoms.
Coronary computed tomography angiography	Looks at blood flow through the coronary arteries. This test can help confirm if there is coronary heart disease.
Invasive coronary angiography	Allows healthcare providers to study blood flow through the heart and coronary arteries. This test can help accurately identify coronary heart disease and determine whether surgery or other procedures might relieve angina symptoms.
Provocation test	This can help diagnose vasospastic and microvascular angina. Can be used during invasive coronary angiography to determine whether a chemical that causes angina symptoms can cause the coronary arteries to spasm.

Some groups especially women and older adults report atypical symptoms that can include dyspnoea, nausea and/or fatigue. This presentation is referred to as the 'angina equivalent' (Hagler et al. 2023).

MANAGEMENT

Angina is a symptom, suggesting that an individual has an underlying obstructive coronary artery disease. Investigations are undertaken to confirm the severity as well as the extent of the underlying coronary artery disease. This will enable management strategies to be developed and to optimise cardiovascular risk reduction. A significant proportion of those people with chest pain will not have angina and the initial assessment should aim to try to identify any alternative diagnoses for these patients at an early stage (SIGN 2018). Treatment may include antiplatelet drugs, nitrates, beta-blockers, calcium channel blockers, angiotensin-converting enzyme inhibitors, statins and coronary angioplasty or coronary artery bypass graft surgery.

Decisions about treatment interventions must be made with the patient where possible and options will take into account the type of angina the person has, symptoms, test results and the risk of complications. To reiterate, unstable angina is a medical emergency that requires immediate treatment in a hospital.

If the person's angina is stable and their symptoms are not getting worse, the condition may be managed with a focus on heart-healthy lifestyle changes along with a pharmacological approach. If lifestyle changes and medicines cannot manage the angina, medical procedures may be required to improve blood flow and relieve symptoms. Treatments for angina usually involve the following two approaches:

- Increasing blood flow to the heart muscle.
- Reducing the heart's workload.

PHARMACOLOGICAL INTERVENTIONS

Fast-acting medicines can be prescribed to manage angina events and relieve pain. Other medication, also prescribed, can be used to help manage angina long term. The choice of medicines depends on what type of angina the person has (see Table 6.4).

Table 6.4 Some pharmacological approaches to angina

Beta-blockers	Nitrates (such as glyceryl trinitrate [GTN])	Calcium channel blockers
Help the heart beat slower and with less force. These medicines may help relieve angina. Side effects can include headache, dizziness and gastrointestinal disturbances. If the person has vasospastic angina, beta-blockers may make the angina worse.	These medications dilate and relax blood vessels. This lowers the heart's workload as well as increases blood flow to the heart muscle. If beta-blockers are unsuitable, long-acting nitrates are the preferred alternative. Nitrate pills (GTN) (see also Box 6.1) or sprays act quickly and can relieve pain during an angina event. Taking nitrates right before an activity that usually triggers angina may help delay or avoid an angina event. Long-acting nitrates are available as pills or skin patches (topical). In hospital settings, for chest pain, intravenous nitrates are administered to relieve pain associated with angina, acting as quickly as possible. Side effects of nitrates can include headache and dizziness.	Calcium channel blockers relax the muscle cells of the heart and blood vessels. If the person is not suited to beta-blockers or nitrates, calcium channel blockers may be another option to relieve symptoms. For vasospastic angina, calcium channel blockers are usually prescribed which avoids giving beta-blockers. Side effects of calcium channel blockers can include headache, drowsiness, gastrointestinal disturbances and ankle oedema.

Source: Adapted from Hagler et al. (2023); British Heart Foundation (2017b,c).

BOX 6.1   GLYCERYL TRINITRATE

Glyceryl trinitrate (GTN) administered sublingually has a rapid onset within 60 seconds lasting for 5–30 minutes (Joint National Formulary).

Safe storage and care of medication for patients taking sublingual GTN tablets:

- Tablets have a short shelf life and deteriorate as soon as the bottle is opened.
- Date when the bottle was opened and discard when expired.
- Refrain from hoarding several open bottles.
- Keep the bottle tightly sealed to protect from the air.

Metered aerosol GTN spray

This preparation is sprayed under the tongue. Absorption is quick and very effective, the area under the tongue is highly vascular and efficient in absorbing the drug rapidly. This preparation is commonly used in acute care settings, for example, urgent care centres and emergency departments.

Transdermal patches of GTN

In patients requiring a constant dose of GTN, patches may be prescribed. The impregnated GTN provides a time-released method of dosing. GTN transdermal patches:

- If appropriate, shave the area where the pad is to be applied.
- Apply a new patch first and then remove the old patch.
- Avoid touching the patch or getting any adhesive on fingers.
- Avoid placing a pad on skin that is irritated or damaged, i.e. scar or in between skin folds.
- Apply a patch on upper arms or chest.
- Remove the used patch and dispose of safely as residual medication may harm others or pets.

GTN ointment

An ointment preparation is applied to the skin every three to four hours as required. This may be applied to the skin of the chest, arm or thigh, the ointment is then covered with surgical tape.

Parenteral (IV) GTN

Administered only in an acute care setting, providing continuous blood pressure and ECG monitoring. Indicated for use if the patient is in a serious clinical condition.

Source: Adapted from Joint National Formulary, Hill (2023) and Hagler et al. (2023).

Other medications may also be prescribed that are used as prophylaxis against myocardial infarction, stroke and other cardiac events (see Table 6.5).

Ranolazine, an anti-angina medication, may be prescribed to prevent angina symptoms from occurring as often. When given with other angina medication, it can also increase the amount of physical activity undertaken without triggering angina. Side effects may include dizziness, headache, constipation and nausea.

Table 6.5 Pharmacological medication: prophylaxis

Medication	Discussion
Antiplatelet medicines	Prevent thrombus formation. In stable or unstable angina, may need aspirin to lower the risks of complications of heart disease. Maybe prescribed a combination of aspirin with platelet inhibitors (i.e. clopidogrel).
Anticoagulant medicines	Also called blood thinners, for example, heparin, slow down clotting and lower risks of blood clots and future complications.
Statins	Prevent plaque from forming and can slow down coronary heart disease. Can also relieve blood vessel spasms or inflammation, lowering the risk of complications after emergency treatment.

Source: Adapted from Bunce, Ray, and Patel (2023), Hill (2023) and Hagler et al. (2023).

OTHER INTERVENTIONS

If lifestyle changes and medicines are unsuccessful in managing the person's angina, other medical procedures may be required to treat the underlying medical condition.

Coronary artery bypass grafting may help treat coronary heart disease and relieve angina. CABG can improve blood flow to the heart, relieve chest pain and help prevent a he art attack.

Percutaneous coronary intervention, also known as coronary angioplasty, can open narrowed or blocked blood vessels that supply blood to the heart (see Figure 6.3). This procedure requires cardiac catheterisation. A stent may be inserted in the artery to help keep the artery open. Combining PCI with certain medicines that widen coronary arteries may help relieve vasospastic angina.

HEALTH TEACHING

It is important for individuals with chronic stable angina to work closely with those who offer care and support to develop a personalised treatment plan, as this condition can be effectively managed, the goal is to reduce symptoms, improve quality of life and prevent heart-related complications.

To prevent angina, there may be a need to adopt healthier lifestyle changes to lower the risk of heart disease, the most common cause of angina. Heart-healthy lifestyle changes include choosing a heart-healthy eating pattern (the Eatwell Guide; Office for Health Improvement and Disparities 2023) being physically active aiming for a healthy weight, quitting smoking and not misusing drugs, managing stress and getting enough good-quality sleep.

Clare (2019) discusses issues to consider on discharge if the patient has been admitted and treated in the hospital. The patient should be advised to call an ambulance if they have angina symptoms that last for more than 10 minutes and have not been relieved by rest or their usual medication. Patients should also be referred to the hospital cardiac rehabilitation programme (NICE 2020). Cardiac rehabilitation is a structured programme of exercise and health promotion, undertaken as a group activity under the supervision of a healthcare professional. The programme includes teaching sessions by dietitians and other health professionals.

For people who have been diagnosed with unstable angina, they will require specific information on self-management. Self-management programmes teach patients skills such as:

- Staging and spacing activities
- Taking appropriate rest

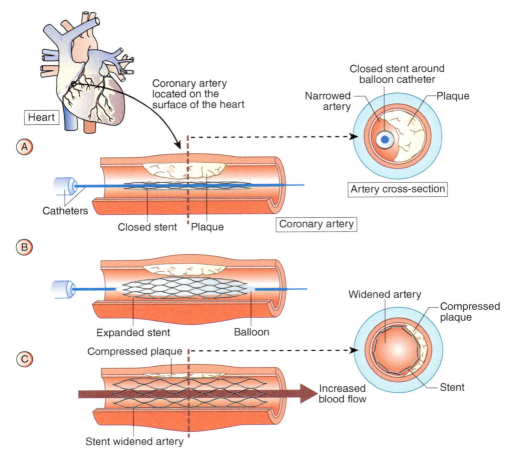

FIGURE 6.3 Percutaneous coronary intervention

- Taking exercise
- Healthy diet
- Managing pain and fatigue
- Dealing with depression or anger
- Communicating with family, friends and healthcare professionals

CONCLUSION

Angina is a symptom rather than a disease itself and typically presents as chest pain or discomfort. It occurs when there is reduced blood flow to the heart muscle due to narrowed coronary arteries. Angina is often a sign of underlying heart disease, such as coronary artery disease. It serves as an important clinical indicator of compromised blood flow to the heart muscle. The clinical presentation of angina can vary; however, there are a number of common features.

Understanding the clinical presentation of angina, its various forms (such as stable and unstable angina) and the associated risk factors is essential for timely diagnosis and management. Recognising the triggers and alleviating factors of angina, as well as the potential for atypical symptoms, is crucial in clinical practice. It is also important to distinguish between stable angina, which can often be managed with lifestyle modifications and medication and unstable angina, which requires immediate intervention due to its association with a higher risk of myocardial infarction.

Those who provide care and support to people with angina must remain vigilant in assessing patients presenting with chest pain or discomfort, consider their medical history, risk factors and the results of diagnostic tests. Accurate diagnosis and early intervention can significantly reduce the risk of adverse cardiovascular events, improve patients' quality of life and enhance long-term outcomes.

GLOSSARY OF TERMS

Angina pectoris: Commonly referred to as angina, a medical term used to describe chest pain or discomfort caused by reduced blood flow to the heart muscle.

Antiplatelet agents: Antiplatelet agents, such as aspirin, help prevent blood clot formation in the arteries, often used in the treatment of angina.

Atherosclerosis: The process of plaque buildup in the arteries, including the coronary arteries, leading to narrowing and reduced blood flow.

Beta-blockers: A class of medications used to manage angina by reducing the heart's workload and oxygen demand.

Cardiac catheterisation: A procedure whereby a thin, flexible tube (catheter) is inserted into a blood vessel and guided to the heart to assess coronary artery blockages and perform interventions such as angioplasty and stent placement.

Coronary artery disease: A condition in which the coronary arteries become narrowed or blocked due to the buildup of plaque.

Ischaemia: A condition where there is a reduced blood supply to an organ or tissue, often due to a blocked or narrowed artery. In the context of angina, it refers to inadequate blood flow to the heart muscle.

Microvascular angina: Also known as cardiac syndrome X, a type of angina in which the small blood vessels in the heart (microvessels) do not function properly, leading to chest pain.

Myocardial infarction: A medical term for a heart attack. It occurs when there is a complete blockage of blood flow to a portion of the heart muscle, leading to tissue damage.

Risk factors: Characteristics or behaviours that increase the likelihood of developing angina or coronary artery disease. Common risk factors include smoking, high blood pressure, high cholesterol, diabetes and family history.

Stable angina: A predictable pattern of chest pain or discomfort occurring with specific triggers, such as physical exertion or stress, usually resolves with rest or medication.

Stent: A small, tube-like medical device made of metal or fabric used to treat various medical conditions, primarily in blood vessels and hollow organs. Designed to provide support, maintain patency and improve blood flow in narrowed or blocked vessels or passages in the body. Commonly used in the treatment of cardiovascular conditions.

Unstable angina: A more serious and unpredictable form of angina. Can occur at rest or with minimal exertion, last longer and may not respond well to medication. It is considered a medical emergency.

Variant (Prinzmetal's): A rare type of angina caused by temporary spasms in the coronary arteries, leading to reduced blood flow to the heart. It can occur at rest and often responds well to medications that relax the arteries.

MULTIPLE CHOICE QUESTIONS

1. What is angina?
   a) A form of arrhythmia
   b) A type of heart attack
   c) A symptom of reduced blood flow to the heart
   d) A lung condition

2. Which of the following is a common symptom of angina?
   a) Shortness of breath
   b) Abdominal pain
   c) Knee pain
   d) Earache

3. What is stable angina?
   a) Angina that occurs suddenly at rest
   b) Angina that is consistently severe
   c) Predictable angina triggered by exertion or stress
   d) Angina with no clear cause

4. Unstable angina is considered:
   a) A medical emergency
   b) A non-serious condition
   c) Similar to stable angina
   d) A chronic condition

5. Nitroglycerine (GTN) is commonly used to:
   a) Increase blood pressure
   b) Relieve angina symptoms
   c) Lower cholesterol levels
   d) Treat diabetes

6. What is the primary goal of angina management?
   a) Cure the underlying heart disease
   b) Prevent all chest pain
   c) Control symptoms and reduce the risk of heart attack
   d) Increase physical activity

7. Which type of angina can occur suddenly, even at rest?
   a) Stable angina
   b) Variant angina
   c) Microvascular angina
   d) Exertional angina

8. Microvascular angina primarily affects which blood vessels?
   a) The main coronary arteries
   b) Large arteries throughout the body
   c) Small blood vessels in the heart
   d) Arteries in the legs

9. Which of the following is a typical trigger for angina symptoms?
   a) Warm weather
   b) Emotional stress
   c) Standing still
   d) Caffeine consumption

10. Which of the following statements about angina is true?
    a) Angina is a condition of the lungs.
    b) All chest pain is angina.
    c) Angina is always a medical emergency.
    d) Angina can be a symptom of underlying heart disease.

REFERENCES

Ashelford, S. and Taylor, V. (2023). Principles of pathophysiology (Chapter 5). In: *The Advanced Practitioner* (eds. I. Peate, S. Diamond-Fox, and B. Hill). Oxford: Wiley.

Bickley, L.S., Szilagyi, P.G., and Hoffman, R.M. (2023). *Bate's Guide to Physical Examination and History Taking*, 13e. Philadelphia: Wolters Kluwer.

British Heart Foundation (2017a). https://www.bhf.org.uk/-/media/files/information-and-support/publications/medical-information-sheets/microvascular_angina_mis_0917.pdf?rev=66d2e67c4668435abbbb4be825a22f63 (accessed October 2023).

British Heart Foundation (2017b). Angina and living life to the full. https://www.bhf.org.uk/-/media/files/information-and-support/publications/heart-conditions/his6_1217_angina_a6.pdf?rev=d296bed440054cdf944a75e3c8e5f147 (accessed October 2023).

British Heart Foundation (2017c). Medicines for my heart. https://www.bhf.org.uk/-/media/files/information-and-support/publications/treatments-for-heart-conditions/bhf_his17_medicines_0817_a6.pdf?rev=cd286757b8bb49cdbacd1079f8fb00b9 (accessed October 2023).

Bunce, N.H., Ray, R., and Patel, H. (2023). Cardiology (Chapter 30). In: *Kumar and Clark's Clinical Medicine*, 10e. (eds. A. Feather, D. Randall, and M. Waterhouse). London: Elsevier.

Clare, C. (2019). Cardiovascular disorders (Chapter 29). In: *Learning to Care* (ed. I. Peate). London: Elsevier.

Ford, T.J. and Berry, C. (2020). Angina: contemporary diagnosis and management. *Heart* 106 (5): 387–398. doi:10.1136/heartjnl-2018-314661.

Hagler, D., Harding, M.M., Kwong, J. et al. (2023). *Lewis's Medical-Surgical Nursing*, 12e. Philadelphia: Elsevier.

Hill, B. (2023). Angina (Chapter 20). In: *Long Term Conditions at a Glance* (eds. A. Mitchell, B. Hill, and I. Peate). Hoboken: Blackwell Publishing.

Joint National Formulary. Glyceryl trinitrate. https://www.nice.org.uk/bnf-uk-only (accessed September 2024).

Menzies-Gow, E. (2019). Nursing patients with cardiovascular disorders (Chapter 3). In: *Alexander's Nursing Practice*, 5e (ed. I. Peate). Edinburgh: Churchill Livingston.

National Institute for Health and Care Excellence (2016). Stable angina: management. https://www.nice.org.uk/guidance/cg126/resources/stable-angina-management-pdf-35109453262021 (accessed October 2023).

National Institute for Health and Care Excellence (2020). Acute coronary syndromes. NICE guideline 185. https://www.nice.org.uk/guidance/ng185 (accessed October 2023).

Office for Health Improvement and Disparities (2023). Healthy eating: applying all our health. https://www.gov.uk/government/publications/healthy-eating-applying-all-our-health (accessed October 2023).

Raleigh, V. (2023). The health of people from ethnic minority groups in England. https://www.kingsfund.org.uk/publications/health-people-ethnic-minority-groups-england#cvd (accessed October 2023).

Sardella, G. and Mancone, M. (2018). Invasive functional test in patients with angina and suspected CAD. *Journal of the American Journal of Cardiology* 72 (23): 2856–2858.

Scottish Intercollegiate Guidelines Network (2018). Management of stable angina. https://www.sign.ac.uk/media/1461/qrg151.pdf (accessed October 2023).

Hypertension

CHAPTER 7

Hypertension is the leading known cause of disability and premature death in the UK, primarily through stroke, heart attack and heart disease. One in three adults in the UK has high hypertension and every day 350 people have a preventable stroke or heart attack caused by the condition. Hypertension is a serious health concern.

Hypertension is defined as persistently raised arterial blood pressure (BP). There is no natural cut-off point above which 'hypertension' definitively exists; any increase in BP may be associated with an increase in renal or cardiovascular disease risk. The current standard threshold for suspecting hypertension is a clinic systolic BP sustained at or above 140 mmHg, or a diastolic BP sustained at or above 90 mmHg or both (National Institute for Health and Care Excellence [NICE] 2020).

PRIMARY AND SECONDARY HYPERTENSION

Hypertension (BP of 140/90 mmHg or greater) can be either primary hypertension, with no single known cause, or secondary hypertension, which means it is related to another factor such as kidney disease (NICE 2020).

Primary hypertension, also called essential hypertension, is the most common form of high BP. Typically, it develops gradually over time and often has no identifiable cause. There are several risk factors and contributing factors that may increase the likelihood of primary hypertension, including genetics, age, lifestyle factors and stress. Secondary hypertension is less common and is caused by an underlying medical condition or medication. Unlike primary hypertension, secondary hypertension often has a specific identifiable cause. Some common causes and contributing factors of secondary hypertension may include renal disorders, hormonal disorders, medications, sleep apnoea and adrenal gland tumours (Blanchflower and Peate 2021).

If hypertension is prolonged, the heart will have an increased workload to maintain circulation, and greater stress will be exerted on the blood vessel walls; cardiac ischaemia may follow.

BLOOD PRESSURE

Each time the heart beats, it contracts, pumping blood into the arteries. The blood is transported to every part of the body, providing it with the energy and oxygen it needs, and a certain amount of pressure is needed to move the blood around the body. When the blood moves along the artery, it exerts pressure against the sides of the blood vessels. The force of this pushing is BP. The pressure is at its highest when the heart beats. This is called the systolic pressure (top number) and this should be around 120 or less. The pressure is at its lowest when the heart relaxes (rests) in between beats. This is called the diastolic pressure (bottom number) and this should be around 80 or less. BP is therefore expressed as two numbers, systolic and diastolic. BP is measured in 'millimetres of mercury' (mmHg). When the BP is measured, it will be written as two numbers. If, for example, the reading is 120/80 mmHg, the BP is said to be '120 over 80'. BP is not usually something that you feel or notice. Table 7.1 demonstrates what different readings can mean.

Table 7.1 Blood pressure (BP) readings and what they might mean

BP reading	What this means	What needs to be done
Less than 120 over 80	The BP is normal.	Re-check in 5 years. Maintain a healthy lifestyle to keep the BP at this level.
Between 121 over 81 and 139 over 89	The BP is a little higher than it should be. There may be a risk of developing hypertension in later life; steps should be taken to try to lower it.	Re-check in a year. Make healthy lifestyle changes.
140 over 90, or higher (over a number of weeks)	This is classed as hypertension.	Lifestyle changes are needed. Patient should see general practitioner or practice nurse and take any medicines prescribed.

Source: Adapted from British Heart Foundation (2023a).

The BP naturally goes up and down throughout the day and night, it is normal for it to go up while a person is mobile. It is when the overall BP is constantly high, even when at rest, that something needs to be done about it, as the heart is working harder when pumping blood around the body.

Box 7.1 discusses blood pressure.

BOX 7.1 BLOOD PRESSURE

Heart contraction (systolic pressure): The heart pumps to circulate blood. When the heart contracts, it pushes blood out into the arteries. This force generates the higher number in the BP reading (systolic pressure). It represents the maximum pressure exerted on artery walls during a heartbeat.

Heart relaxation (diastolic pressure): After each heartbeat, the heart relaxes momentarily. During this phase, the pressure in the arteries decreases. The lower number in the BP reading is called diastolic pressure. It represents the minimum pressure in the arteries when the heart is at rest.

Blood vessel resistance: BP is influenced by the resistance the blood encounters as it flows through the arteries. The narrower the arteries or the greater the resistance, the higher the BP. Factors such as the diameter of blood vessels, their elasticity and the thickness of blood can affect this resistance.

Regulation: The body regulates BP through a complex system that involves the nervous system, hormones and feedback mechanisms. The autonomic nervous system plays a vital role in adjusting BP. The sympathetic nervous system increases heart rate and narrows blood vessels, leading to hypertension, while the parasympathetic nervous system does the opposite.

Hormones: Hormones such as adrenaline and aldosterone can also influence BP. Adrenaline, for example, can increase heart rate and contractility, leading to hypertension during stress or excitement. Aldosterone regulates salt and water balance, affecting blood volume and, as such, BP.

Baroreceptor reflex: Specialised sensors, baroreceptors are located in the walls of certain blood vessels, such as the carotid arteries and the aorta, continuously monitoring BP. They send signals to the brain, which responds by adjusting heart rate, blood vessel diameter and other factors to maintain BP within a narrow range.

THE CARDIAC CYCLE

The cardiac cycle reflects a series of electrical and mechanical events occurring throughout each heartbeat, resulting in the ejection of blood from the right and left ventricles. It can be separated into distinct phases: the first phase diastole where the heart is in a relaxed state allowing it to fill with blood; the second phase systole where the myocardium is contracting. The contraction of the atria shortly followed by the contraction of the ventricles in conjunction with the heart valves ensures a unidirectional flow of blood through the heart; this results in systolic ejection of blood into the systemic and pulmonary circulations (Sinnott 2022). See Figure 7.1, the cardiac cycle.

The equation 'Blood pressure = cardiac output × peripheral vascular resistance (BP = CO × PVR)' represents the basic physiological relationship between BP, CO and PVR. It is used to explain how changes in these factors can influence BP. See Box 7.2.

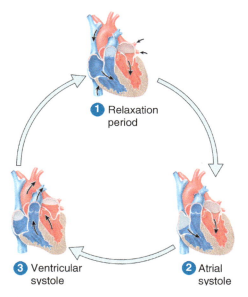

FIGURE 7.1 The cardiac cycle

BOX 7.2 — HAEMODYNAMIC EQUATION (BLOOD PRESSURE EQUATION)

'Blood pressure = cardiac output × peripheral vascular resistance (BP = CO × PVR)'

Suppose an individual's CO is 5 L/min^{-1} and their peripheral vascular resistance (PVR) is 20 units (the units can vary depending on the measurement method). To calculate their BP:

$$BP = CO \times PVR$$
$$BP = 5\,L/min^{-1} \times 20\ units$$
$$BP = 100\ units\ of\ blood\ pressure\ (mmHg,\ for\ example)$$

In this example, the individual's BP would be 100 units of BP, which could be measured in mmHg.

PATHOPHYSIOLOGICAL CHANGES ASSOCIATED WITH HYPERTENSION

Those with arterial hypertension may have an increase in cardiac output, an increase in systemic vascular resistance or both. Hypertension usually begins with the narrowing of the small arteries and arterioles throughout the body. This narrowing is mainly due to the blood vessels constricting or becoming stiffer. When the blood vessels are narrow, this increases the resistance that the heart has to overcome to pump blood through them. To overcome this increased resistance, the heart pumps harder and faster, causing an increased cardiac output. More blood is pumped per minute.

The combination of narrowed blood vessels, increased resistance and higher cardiac output causes elevated BP. Elevated BP can damage various organs over time (Hill 2023).

EPIDEMIOLOGY

Hypertension is the leading modifiable risk factor for heart and circulatory disease in the UK. There are an estimated 28% of adults in the UK who have hypertension; this equates to around 15 million adults and at least half of them are not receiving effective treatment. Over 10 million people in the UK have been diagnosed with hypertension by their GP; up to 4.8 million adults, therefore, could be undiagnosed. It is estimated in the UK, that 6–8 million people are living with undiagnosed or uncontrolled hypertension (British Heart Foundation 2023b).

RISK FACTORS

There are a number of modifiable and non-modifiable factors that can increase the risk of developing hypertension. See Table 7.2.

The World Health Organization (WHO 2021) discusses hypertension, and Public Health England (2017) has provided a professional resource that outlines how healthcare providers can reduce the population average BP through improved prevention, detection and management, see below:

NON-MODIFIABLE RISK FACTORS

AGE

In the UK, as in other developed nations, BP tends to rise with age. In England, the increase in average systolic pressure between ages 16–24 years and 75 years and above is just under 20 mmHg. It is thought that this reflects the length of time that people are exposed to modifiable lifestyle risk factors.

Table 7.2 Modifiable and non-modifiable risk factors associated with hypertension (Public Health England 2017)

Modifiable	Non-modifiable
Excess dietary salt	Age
Poor diet and obesity	Ethnicity
Excess alcohol consumption	Genetics
Lack of physical activity	Gender
Deprivation and socioeconomic status	
Mental health and stress	

GENDER

Health Survey for England demonstrates that for any given age up to around 65 years, women tend to have lower BP than men. Between 65 and 74 years of age, women tend to have higher BP. With regards to prevalence, in England, the proportion of the population with hypertension increased from 5% of men and 1% of women aged 16–24 years to 58% in men and women aged 65–74 years.

ETHNICITY

People who are from Black African and Black Caribbean ethnic groups in England have a higher risk of hypertension than the general population, although any differences in hypertension between other ethnic groups are not always apparent. Ethnic groups, for example, South Asian, Black African and Black Caribbean communities, are more prone to developing type 2 diabetes, which also increases the risk of having hypertension.

GENETICS

Genetic factors play some role in hypertension, heart disease and other related conditions.

MODIFIABLE RISK FACTORS

There are a number of environmental risk factors that are driving the epidemic of cardiovascular disease. Health professionals and local authorities are encouraged to raise awareness of these factors and support people to make healthy lifestyle changes.

EXCESS DIETARY SALT

Excess dietary salt is one of the most important modifiable risk factors for hypertension. A high salt diet disrupts the natural sodium balance in the body. This causes fluid retention, increasing the pressure exerted by the blood against blood vessel walls.

Work on salt reduction began in the UK in 2004 following advice from the Scientific Advisory Committee on Nutrition (SACN); it was recommended that the population average salt intake should be reduced to 6 g per day to reduce the risk of hypertension and hence cardiovascular disease (Public Health England 2020).

OBESITY

It is not just a diet that is high in salt that can increase the risk of hypertension. Eating a diet high in calories and fat, especially saturated fat and low in fruit and vegetables increases the risk of becoming overweight or obese. Obese men are more than twice as likely to develop hypertension and obese women are three times more likely. There is a strong and direct relationship between excess weight and hypertension.

EXCESS ALCOHOL CONSUMPTION

Alcohol has been identified as a causal factor in more than 60 medical conditions, including hypertension. Heavy habitual consumption of alcohol is linked to raised BP. BP rises, in some cases to dangerous levels, when large amounts of alcohol are consumed – particularly when binge-drinking.

LACK OF PHYSICAL ACTIVITY

Those who do not take enough aerobic exercise are more likely to have or to develop hypertension. People in the UK are around 20% less active now than in the 1960s. If current trends continue, by 2030 we will be 35% less active.

IMPACT OF DEPRIVATION AND SOCIOECONOMIC STATUS

The burden of hypertension is greatest among individuals from low-income households and those living in deprived areas. People from the most deprived areas in England are more likely than the least deprived to have hypertension. These inequalities are wider still for outcomes of hypertension such as stroke and coronary heart disease.

MENTAL HEALTH

Many forms of mental health issues can affect heart disease. Anxiety and stress can increase hormones such as adrenaline and cortisol, which impact BP and heart rate.

It is also thought that people who are stressed may deal with that stress by engaging in unhealthy eating habits, as well as smoking and drinking, and this increases their risk of having hypertension.

CLINICAL PRESENTATION

Hypertension is usually asymptomatic until complications develop in target organs. Dizziness, facial flushing, headache, fatigue, epistaxis and nervousness are not typically caused by uncomplicated hypertension. Severe hypertension (typically defined as systolic BP ≥ 180 mmHg and/or diastolic BP ≥ 120 mmHg) can be asymptomatic (hypertensive urgency). When severe hypertension causes severe cardiovascular, neurological, renal and retinal symptoms, it is referred to as a hypertensive emergency (see Figure 7.2).

Undiagnosed or uncontrolled hypertension can lead to serious health problems such as:

ANEURYSM

Aortic aneurysms are balloon-like bulges occurring in the aorta. The aorta has thick walls that are able to sustain normal BP. However, certain medical problems, genetic conditions and trauma can damage or weaken these walls. The force of blood pushing against the weakened or injured walls can result in an aneurysm.

STROKE

A stroke can occur when blood flow to the brain is blocked or there is a sudden haemorrhage in the brain. A stroke that occurs because the blood flow to the brain is blocked is known as ischaemic stroke. When a stroke occurs because of sudden bleeding in the brain it is called a haemorrhagic stroke.

Clinical Presentation 119

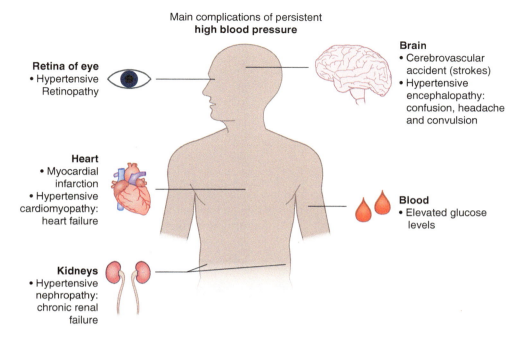

FIGURE 7.2 Complications of hypertension. *Source:* Adapted from Public Health England (2017).

CHRONIC KIDNEY DISEASE

Chronic kidney disease indicates the kidneys are damaged and are unable to filter blood as they should. The main risk factors for developing kidney disease are diabetes, hypertension, heart disease and a family history of kidney failure.

EYE DAMAGE

Hypertension can damage blood vessels in the retina. The retina is the layer of tissue at the back part of the eye; it changes light and images that enter the eye into nerve signals that are sent to the brain. The higher the BP and the longer it has been high, then the more severe the damage is likely to be.

MYOCARDIAL INFARCTION

Myocardial infarction is a serious medical emergency in which the supply of blood to the heart is suddenly blocked, usually by a blood clot. History of hypertension is a frequent finding in patients with myocardial infarction.

HEART FAILURE

Heart failure is a condition that develops when the heart does not pump enough blood for the body's needs.

PERIPHERAL ARTERY DISEASE

Peripheral artery disease is caused by atherosclerosis, or plaque buildup, that reduces the flow of blood in peripheral arteries.

VASCULAR DEMENTIA

Vascular dementia develops when the blood vessels in the brain are damaged by other health conditions. This damage keeps the brain from getting the oxygen it needs. Vascular diseases such as atherosclerosis or hypertension contribute to dementia.

BLOOD PRESSURE MEASUREMENT

The initial step in diagnosing hypertension involves taking multiple BP measurements on different occasions. BP is measured using a sphygmomanometer (with a BP cuff) and a stethoscope or an automated BP monitor. Box 7.3 outlines the procedure for assessing BP using a sphygmomanometer.

BOX 7.3 BLOOD PRESSURE MEASUREMENT

In order to take a patient's BP, you will need (see Figure 7.3):

- Manual sphygmomanometer with a suitable size cuff
- Stethoscope

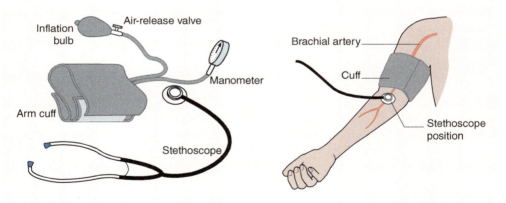

FIGURE 7.3 Sphygmomanometer and stethoscope. *Source:* Clare (2021). With permission of John Wiley & Sons.

FIGURE 7.4 Correct positioning of cuff

1. Place the cuff of the sphygmomanometer around the arm with the centre of the bladder over the brachial artery. The bladder of the cuff should be large enough to circle 80% of the arm but not more than 100% (see Figure 7.4).
2. Estimate the systolic pressure by feeling the brachial pulse with two or three fingers and inflating the cuff until the pulse disappears. Remember to watch the reading on the sphygmomanometer so that you know at what point the pulse disappears. Release the pressure in the cuff. Estimating the systolic pressure ensures that you do not unnecessarily overinflate the cuff when measuring the BP, thus avoiding unnecessary distress and potential harm.

3. Inflate the cuff again until the pressure is approximately 30 mmHg above the point that you estimated the systolic pressure to be. Inflating the cuff 30 mmHg above ensures a safe margin while avoiding unnecessary overinflation.
4. Place the diaphragm of the stethoscope on the place where the brachial pulse was palpated. Some people place the diaphragm before inflating the cuff – this is acceptable so long as no part of the stethoscope is underneath any part of the cuff.
5. Deflate the cuff at a rate of 2–3 mmHg per second until you hear a tapping sound (first Korotkoff sound). This is systolic pressure – make a mental note of that number.
6. Continue to deflate the cuff at a rate of 2–3 mmHg per second until the tapping sound disappears (fifth Korotkoff sound). This is the diastolic pressure – make a mental note of that number.
7. Both the systolic and diastolic should be measured to the nearest 2 mmHg.
8. Deflate the cuff fully and record the systolic and diastolic on the appropriate documentation.

Source: Adapted from Clare (2021).

Blood pressure should be measured in a relaxed, temperate setting, having relaxed for at least five minutes, with the person quiet and seated, their arm outstretched. Ensure that the patient is comfortable and that no tight clothing is restricting the arm; support the arm at the level of the heart, for instance, by using a pillow.

The BP is measured in both arms using an appropriate cuff size. If the difference in readings between arms is more than 15 mmHg, repeat the measurements. If the difference in readings between arms remains more than 15 mmHg on the second measurement, measure subsequent BPs in the arm with the higher reading.

In those with symptoms of postural hypotension (falls or postural dizziness), measure BP with the person either supine or seated. Measure BP again with the person standing for at least one minute before measurement. If the systolic BP falls by 20 mmHg or more when the person is standing, measure subsequent BPs with the person standing.

If BP measured in the clinic is 140/90 mmHg or higher, take a second measurement during the consultation. If the second measurement is substantially different from the first, take a third measurement. Record the lower of the last two measurements as the clinic BP.

If the person's BP is between 140/90 and 180/120 mmHg, offer ambulatory BP monitoring to confirm the diagnosis of hypertension. If ambulatory BP monitoring is unsuitable or the person is unable to tolerate it, offer home BP monitoring.

NICE (2022) suggests that while waiting for confirmation of a diagnosis of hypertension, carry out investigations for target organ damage, followed by a formal assessment of the person's cardiovascular risk. Confirm the diagnosis of hypertension in people with a clinical BP of 140/90 mmHg or higher and a daytime average or home BP monitoring average of 135/85 mmHg or higher. Suspect secondary hypertension in people under the age of 40 years or those who present with accelerated hypertension or where features in the history, examination or investigations point to an underlying cause. Consider current medication as a possible cause for raised BP.

WHITE COAT SYNDROME

Also known as white coat hypertension or white coat effect is a phenomenon in which an individual's BP readings are higher when taken in a medical or clinical setting (such as a GP surgery or hospital) than when measured outside that environment, such as at home. This rise in BP is often attributed to the anxiety, stress or nervousness that some people experience when they visit the GP or the hospital. Multiple readings may be necessary to confirm a diagnosis.

CLINICAL INVESTIGATIONS AND DIAGNOSIS

The diagnosis of hypertension is typically made through a series of BP measurements and assessments. To make a diagnosis of hypertension, there is a need for two or more BP readings at separate medical appointments.

Medical history is taken to determine any risk factors and to obtain general information about the person's health, for example, their eating habits, physical activity level and family's health history. This information will help to develop a treatment plan for the individual and decide if there is a need for the person to undergo any investigations.

A number of investigations may be required depending on the needs of the individual. Target organs that are subject to damage as a result of hypertension are assessed, for example (NICE 2022):

- Test for haematuria.

- Arrange measurement of urine albumin: creatinine ratio (to test for the presence of protein in the urine).

- HbA1C (to test for diabetes).

- Electrolytes, creatinine and estimated glomerular filtration rate (to test for chronic kidney disease).

- Examine the fundi (for the presence of hypertensive retinopathy).

- Arrange for a 12-lead electrocardiograph to be performed (to assess cardiac function and detect left ventricular hypertrophy).

- Consider the need for specialist investigations in people with signs and symptoms suggesting target organ damage or a secondary cause of hypertension.

- Assess cardiovascular risk.

- Arrange measurement of serum total cholesterol and high-density lipoprotein cholesterol.

- Consider the need for investigations for possible secondary causes of hypertension.

MANAGEMENT

It has been suggested that a patient's knowledge of their own goal BP is linked with improved BP control (NICE 2020). Interventions that aim to improve knowledge of specific BP targets can have an important role in improving BP management (NICE 2020).

People have a right to be involved in making choices about their care. In order for them to make a decision, they need to know what their options are and what might happen if they decide that they do not want any treatment or care; they need to be listened to. When patients feel that they have been heard and respected in the decision-making process, this can lead to stronger trust between the patient and the healthcare provider. Trust is an essential component of the therapeutic patient-provider relationship.

Shared decision-making is a joint process in which a healthcare professional works together with a person to decide on care. It puts the patient at the centre of decisions regarding their own treatment and care, acknowledging their values, preferences and goals. This can ensure that healthcare decisions will align with what matters most to the patient, promoting patient satisfaction and engagement in their care. This means that the healthcare provider discusses the different choices that are available to the patient. It involves choosing tests and treatments that are based both on evidence and on the person's individual preferences, beliefs and values. Care or treatment options have to be explored in full, along with the risks and benefits. The ultimate aim is that patients can reach a decision with their health and social care professional. It can ensure that the person understands the risks, benefits and possible consequences of different options through discussion and information sharing.

When patients are actively involved in the decision-making process, they are more likely to adhere to the chosen treatment plan. This can lead to better health outcomes, as patients are more committed to their care. An open communication approach that takes place when there is shared decision-making between patients and healthcare providers can lead to a better understanding of the patient's medical history and context, reducing the possibility of medical errors.

Respecting a patient's autonomy and their right to make decisions about their own healthcare is a key ethical principle. This principle is upheld by involving patients in choices that affect their health.

No two patients are the same; different patients may have different values, preferences and individual circumstances that affect their treatment decisions; they are unique. Shared decision-making enables the customisation of care plans to suit individual needs, promoting more effective and appropriate care.

ADOPTING A HEALTHY LIFESTYLE

Healthy lifestyle changes are advocated for those who have been diagnosed with hypertension. This can help to lower and control hypertension. Choosing heart-healthy foods combined with a low-salt eating plan can be effective as medicines in lowering hypertension. Aim for a healthy weight, avoid or limit alcohol and stop smoking. Undertake regular physical activity and manage stress. Learning how to manage stress and cope with problems can improve mental and physical health. Get enough good-quality sleep.

MEDICINES

When healthy lifestyle changes alone do not control or lower hypertension, the person may be prescribed anti-hypertensive medications. These medicines act in different ways to lower BP. When prescribing medicines, consideration has to be given to their effect on other conditions the person may have, such as heart disease or kidney disease.

All medications have potential side effects; if a person experiences these, they should discuss this with the general practitioner (GP) or doctor about any concerns regarding the side effects from the medicines. A decision may be made to change the dose or prescribe a new medicine. To manage hypertension, many people need to take two or more medicines.

Some common anti-hypertensive medicines that may be prescribed:

- Angiotensin-converting enzyme (ACE) inhibitors help prevent blood vessels from narrowing.

- Angiotensin II receptor blockers (ARBs) keep blood vessels from narrowing.

- Calcium channel blockers prevent calcium from entering the muscle cells of the heart and blood vessels. This allows blood vessels to relax.

- Diuretics remove extra water and sodium from body, reducing the amount of fluid in the blood. The main diuretic for high BP treatment is thiazide. Diuretics are often used with other high BP medicines, sometimes in one combined pill.

- Beta-blockers help the heart to beat slower and with less force. As a result, the heart pumps less blood through the blood vessels. Beta-blockers are typically used only as a backup option or if the patient has other conditions.

HEALTH TEACHING

The WHO (2023) suggests that the following lifestyle changes can help prevent and lower high BP.

Do:

- Eat more vegetables and fruits.
- Sit less.
- Be more physically active, which can include walking, running, swimming, dancing or activities that build strength, such as lifting weights.
- Get at least 150 minutes per week of moderate-intensity aerobic activity or 75 minutes per week of vigorous aerobic activity.
- Do strength-building exercises two or more days each week.
- Lose weight if overweight or obese.
- Take medicines as prescribed by the healthcare professional.
- Keep appointments with healthcare professionals.

Do not:

- Eat too much salty food (try to stay under 2 g per day).
- Eat foods high in saturated or trans fats.
- Smoke or use tobacco.
- Drink too much alcohol (one drink daily maximum for women, two for men).
- Miss or share medication.

Reducing hypertension can prevent myocardial infarction, stroke and renal damage as well as other health problems. Reduce the risks of hypertension by:

- Reducing and managing stress.
- Regularly checking BP.
- Treating hypertension.
- Managing other medical conditions.

CONCLUSION

Hypertension is often referred to as the 'silent killer' as it typically develops without noticeable symptoms; however, it significantly increases the risk of heart disease, stroke, kidney damage and other health issues.

Hypertension is a prevalent and potentially life-threatening condition that is encountered frequently in clinical practice. Understanding the causes, consequences and management of hypertension is vital for providing excellent patient care. Your role in educating, supporting and monitoring patients with hypertension can make a significant difference in their health outcomes.

GLOSSARY OF TERMS

Aneurysm: A weakened and bulging section of a blood vessel that can be life-threatening if it ruptures.

Antihypertensive medications: Medications prescribed to lower blood pressure, including diuretics, beta-blockers, ACE inhibitors, calcium channel blockers and angiotensin receptor blockers (ARBs).

Atherosclerosis: The buildup of fatty deposits (plaques) in the arteries, contributing to high blood pressure and other cardiovascular problems.

Blood pressure: The force exerted by blood against the walls of arteries as the heart pumps it throughout the circulatory system. It is typically expressed as systolic/diastolic pressure (e.g. 120/80 mmHg).

Cardiac output: The amount of blood the heart pumps per minute, influenced by heart rate and stroke volume.

Diastolic pressure: The lower number in a blood pressure reading, representing the force when the heart is at rest between beats.

Hypertension: A medical condition characterised by consistently elevated blood pressure levels in the arteries, often referred to as high blood pressure.

Lifestyle modifications: Changes in diet, physical activity, stress management and smoking cessation aimed at reducing blood pressure and managing hypertension.

Peripheral artery disease: Reduced blood flow in the arteries of the limbs, often associated with hypertension and characterised by leg pain during walking (claudication).

Peripheral vascular resistance: The resistance encountered by blood flow in small arteries and arterioles throughout the body, a key factor in hypertension.

Primary hypertension (essential hypertension): The most common form of hypertension with no identifiable cause, often related to genetics and lifestyle factors.

Secondary hypertension: High blood pressure resulting from an underlying medical condition or medication, which can be treated by addressing the underlying cause.

Stroke volume: The volume of blood ejected from the heart with each beat.

Systolic pressure: The higher number in a blood pressure reading, representing the force when the heart contracts and pumps blood into the arteries.

Target organ damage: Harmful effects of long-term hypertension on organs such as the heart, kidneys, brain, eyes and blood vessels.

White coat syndrome: A condition where blood pressure readings are higher in a medical setting due to anxiety or stress, but normal in other environments.

MULTIPLE CHOICE QUESTIONS

1. What is hypertension?
   a) Low blood pressure
   b) Normal blood pressure
   c) High blood pressure
   d) Irregular blood pressure

2. What are the two main categories of hypertension?
   a) Primary and secondary
   b) Acute and chronic
   c) Systolic and diastolic
   d) Benign and malignant

3. What is the typical classification for normal blood pressure?
   a) 120/80 mmHg
   b) 140/90 mmHg
   c) 130/80 mmHg
   d) 110/70 mmHg

4. What is systolic blood pressure?
   a) The lower number in a blood pressure reading
   b) The pressure when the heart is at rest
   c) The pressure when the heart contracts
   d) The average blood pressure

5. Which term describes elevated blood pressure readings in a clinical setting due to anxiety or stress?
   a) White coat syndrome
   b) Silent hypertension
   c) Masked hypertension
   d) Secondary hypertension

6. What is the primary cause of primary (essential) hypertension?
   a) Genetic factors
   b) Underlying medical conditions
   c) Medication side effects
   d) Unknown, multifactorial factors

7. Which of the following organ systems is NOT commonly affected by long-term hypertension?
   a) Cardiovascular system
   b) Respiratory system
   c) Kidneys
   d) Eyes

8. Which class of antihypertensive drugs helps the body eliminate excess sodium and fluid?
   a) Beta-blockers
   b) ACE inhibitors
   c) Diuretics
   d) Calcium channel blockers

9. What is the term for the force of blood against arterial walls when the heart is at rest between beats?
   a) Systolic pressure
   b) Diastolic pressure
   c) Peripheral vascular resistance
   d) Cardiac output

10. What is the primary consequence of untreated hypertension?
    a) Weight loss
    b) Vision improvement
    c) Organ damage and disease
    d) Increased physical fitness

REFERENCES

Blanchflower, J. and Peate, I. (2021). The vascular system and associated disorders (Chapter 9). In: *Fundamentals of Applied Pathophysiology*, 4e (ed. I. Peate). Oxford: Wiley.

British Heart Foundation (2023a). High blood pressure (hypertension) https://www.bhf.org.uk/informationsupport/risk-factors/high-blood-pressure#normalbp (accessed September 2024).

British Heart Foundation (2023b). UK factsheet. BHF UK CVD factsheet. https://www.bhf.org.uk/-/media/files/for-professionals/research/heart-statistics/bhf-cvd-statistics-uk-factsheet.pdf?rev=c7ad10c134bd46a4aae483cc8d4b7c16&hash=51068640774D775C4F1DFD525B5F9EBA (accessed October 2023).

Clare, C. (2021). Vital signs. In: *The Nursing Associate's Handbook of Clinical Skills*? (ed. I. Peate). Oxford: Wiley.

Hill, B. (2023). Hypertension (Chapter 40). In: *Long Term Conditions at A Glance* (eds. A. Mitchell, B. Hill, and I. Peate). Oxford: Wiley.

National Institute for Health and Care Excellence (2020). Peripheral arterial disease: diagnosis and management. https://www.nice.org.uk/guidance/cg147 (accessed October 2023).

National Institute for Health and Care Excellence (2022). Hypertension in adults: diagnosis and management. https://www.nice.org.uk/guidance/ng136/resources/hypertension-in-adults-diagnosis-and-management-pdf-66141722710213 (accessed October 2023).

Public Health England (2017). Health matters: combating high blood pressure. https://www.gov.uk/government/publications/health-matters-combating-high-blood-pressure/health-matters-combating-high-blood-pressure (accessed October 2023).

Public Health England (2020). Salt reduction targets for 2024. https://assets.publishing.service.gov.uk/media/5f5618c8d3bf7f4d75de6ff1/2024_salt_reduction_targets_070920-FINAL-1.pdf (accessed October 2023).

Sinnott, P. (2022). Cardiac physiology (Chapter 18). In: *Fundamentals of Critical Care* (eds. I. Peate and B. Hill). Oxford: Wiley.

World Health Organization (2021). Hyper-tension. https://www.who.int/news-room/fact-sheets/detail/hypertension (accessed October 2023).

World Health Organization (2023). Hypertension. https://www.who.int/news-room/fact-sheets/detail/hypertension (accessed October 2023).

CHAPTER 8 Peripheral Arterial Disease

There are many definitions of peripheral arterial disease (PAD). PAD is a term that is used to describe the narrowing or occlusion of the peripheral arteries, involving the blood supply usually to the lower limbs. This causes a reduction in blood flow to the limb that has been affected. The narrowing or occlusion is usually a result of arterial atherosclerotic disease. The majority of patients with this condition are asymptomatic; however, there are some patients who experience intermittent claudication (this is pain that occurs while walking). Chronic limb-threatening ischaemia (previously known as critical limb ischaemia) occurs when there is a reduction in blood flow that is so severe it causes the person pain at rest or loss of tissue (for example, ulceration or gangrene).

Figure 8.1 depicts the main arteries in the leg. They include the femoral artery, deep femoral artery, popliteal artery, posterior tibial artery and anterior tibial artery. These arteries provide a rich supply of oxygenated blood and nutrients to the lower limbs.

PAD is also known as peripheral vascular disease (PVD). Bunce, Ray, and Patel (2023) note that peripheral venous disease includes venous thromboembolic disease, varicose veins and superficial thrombophlebitis. Table 8.1 describes chronic limb-threatening ischaemia and acute limb ischaemia.

NICE (2020) notes that rapid changes in diagnostic methods, endovascular treatments and vascular services that are associated with new specialties in surgery and interventional radiology have caused significant uncertainty and variation in practice.

PATHOPHYSIOLOGICAL CHANGES ASSOCIATED WITH PAD

PAD is a lifelong medical condition; there is no cure for PVD. Once a diagnosis of PAD has been made, ongoing care and treatment will be required, and the person will need to take steps to prevent complications. PAD is a marker for increased risk of cardiovascular events even when it is asymptomatic.

PAD causes leg pain or discomfort, which most commonly occurs on exertion and it resolves after rest (known as intermittent claudication); however, some people have no obvious symptoms even when functional impairment is noticeable on testing. Claudication is a manifestation of exercise-induced reversible ischaemia, similar to angina pectoris.

Those people with PAD are at increased risk of myocardial infarction, ischaemic stroke and death. To reduce the risk of cardiovascular events, guidelines (for example, NICE 2020) recommend the use of antiplatelet therapy and statins for all individuals with symptomatic PAD, along with antihypertensive therapy for those with associated hypertension. ACE inhibitors may also reduce cardiovascular risk in those symptomatic patients with PAD.

Incidence is also high in those with coronary artery disease and in people with diabetes; early diagnosis and management of PAD is therefore important. In the majority of patients with intermittent claudication, their symptoms will remain stable, but approximately 20% will go on and develop increasingly severe symptoms with the development of chronic limb-threatening ischaemia (see Box 8.1).

Pathophysiological Changes Associated with PAD   129

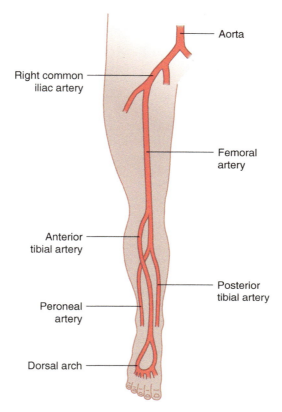

FIGURE 8.1   Lower limb arteries

Table 8.1   Limb ischaemia

Type of ischaemia	Discussion
Chronic limb-threatening ischaemia	Intermittent claudication
	This is the most common clinical symptom associated with PAD and occurs when diminished circulation leads to pain in the lower limbs during walking or exercise that is relieved by rest.
	It occurs when circulation is so severely impaired that there is an imminent risk of limb loss.
	This term describes clinical patterns with threatened limb viability that are related to several factors. It is characterised by chronic, inadequate tissue perfusion at rest and is defined by ischaemic rest pain with or without tissue loss (for example, ulcers, gangrene or infection).
	It represents the end stage of PAD.
Acute limb ischaemia	This is a sudden decrease in limb perfusion that threatens limb viability. In acute limb ischaemia, decreased perfusion and symptoms and signs develop over less than two weeks.

Source: Adapted from the National Institute for Health and Care Excellence (NICE 2020), Farber (2018), and Gerhard-Herman et al. (2017).

| BOX 8.1 | CHRONIC LIMB-THREATENING ISCHAEMIA |

Chronic limb-threatening ischaemia is severely blocked blood flow to one or multiple hands, legs or feet. It causes intense pain, numbness and slow-healing ulcers on the feet, legs or hands. It is a serious condition that increases the person's risk of heart complications, limb amputation and death.

Chronic limb-threatening ischaemia is a severe stage of PAD. PAD occurs when atherosclerotic plaque builds up inside the arteries and restricts blood flow.

It is harder for the muscles and tissues to remain healthy, or to heal, when there is limited blood flow.

Chronic limb-threatening ischaemia is an extremely serious complication that can be challenging to treat. It is considered the most serious form of PAD.

EPIDEMIOLOGY

Gerhard-Herman et al. (2017) estimated that globally there are over 200 million people with PAD. Cea-Soriano et al. (2018), referring to the UK data, found a decreasing incidence and prevalence of symptomatic PAD being diagnosed in primary care. It was suggested that this decline could have been brought about by an increased uptake of secondary prevention strategies. PVD is present in 7% of middle-aged men and 4.5% of middle-aged women; however, the mortality that is associated with co-existing cardiovascular and cerebrovascular disease means that only a proportion of patients with PVD progress to losing their legs (Bunce, Ray, and Patel 2023).

PAD is uncommon in younger people; it increases with age. Evidence from population studies suggests that about 20% of people aged over 60 years have some degree of PAD (NICE 2020).

RISK FACTORS

Risk factors are the same as those for cardiovascular diseases (atherosclerosis), smoking and diabetes mellitus being the strongest. Smoking (or other forms of tobacco use) has been shown to be one of the strongest risk factors for PAD (Mills, Japp, and Robson 2018). Smoking at least doubles the odds of PAD compared with not smoking, and heavier smokers are at increased risk compared with light smokers. People with PAD who continue to smoke are at increased risk of developing claudication and chronic limb-threatening ischaemia; they are twice as likely to need limb amputation compared with someone who stops smoking.

Diabetes mellitus is strongly associated with an increased risk of PAD, particularly in those with more severe, poorly controlled or longstanding diabetes. Evidence suggests outcomes of PAD (such as amputation rates and mortality) are worse in people with diabetes (Rajan et al. 2022). Other factors include:

- Advanced age.
- Hypertension (there is an association between hypertension and PAD).
- Hypercholesterolaemia (total cholesterol is significantly associated with peripheral arterial disease).
- Known atherosclerotic disease elsewhere (such as coronary, carotid, abdominal aorta).
- Chronic kidney disease (particularly in people with end-stage renal disease needing dialysis).

The more risk factors a person has, the risk of having PAD increases.

CLINICAL PRESENTATION

Intermittent claudication is the most common initial symptom of lower limb PAD (NICE 2020). Clinical presentation can vary depending on the severity of the disease.

Chronic limb-threatening ischaemia may present when there is progressive development of a cramp-like pain in the calf, thigh or buttock on walking, which is relieved by resting; there may be unexplained foot or leg pain or non-healing wounds on the lower limb (Hagler et al. 2023; Mitchell 2023). Intermittent claudication is one of the hallmark symptoms of PAD. There are some people who may present with atypical symptoms; they may use terminology such as 'tired', 'giving way', 'sore and hurts', as opposed to describing cramps.

As PAD progresses, the distance that the person can walk without symptoms may decrease and those with severe PAD may experience pain during rest, which reflects irreversible ischaemia. Rest pain is usually worse distally, and it is aggravated by leg elevation (causing pain at night); this lessens when the leg is below heart level.

Skin changes may occur. Patients with PAD may exhibit skin changes in the affected limb, including pallor; the skin may appear pale or blanched when elevated. In severe cases, the skin may appear bluish or mottled due to reduced oxygen supply. Some limbs have a deep red/purple hue (dependent rubor); this occurs due to the arteries in the foot vasodilating, attempting to oxygenate the lower limb adequately, which results in pooling of the arterial blood. This may give the appearance of cellulitis or a well-perfused limb, skin can appear atrophic shiny. The colour remains the same if the limb is elevated or dependent.

The limb may feel cooler to the touch compared to the unaffected limb. As a result of decreased blood flow to the extremities, there may be reduced hair growth on the legs and feet. The patient may have brittle or thickened toenails.

During physical examination, pulses in the affected limb are weak or absent. Common pulse sites to assess include the dorsalis pedis and posterior tibial pulses.

In severe cases of PAD, the patient may develop non-healing wounds or ulcers, often on the toes, feet or legs. These ulcers can become infected and lead to gangrene if not treated promptly (Mitchell, 2023). As a result of chronic lack of blood flow, this may lead to muscle weakness and atrophy in the affected limb.

Some patients may experience numbness or tingling in the legs and feet due to reduced nerve function caused by inadequate blood supply. The affected leg may sweat excessively. This may be due to sympathetic nerve overactivity.

It should be noted that not all patients with PAD will exhibit all of these symptoms, and the severity of symptoms may vary widely. Some people may have mild intermittent claudication; others, however, may present with chronic limb-threatening ischaemia.

If suspected, see the sections on assessment and features of intermittent claudication and critical limb ischaemia.

CLINICAL INVESTIGATIONS AND DIAGNOSIS

Early detection and intervention are essential in managing PAD and preventing complications. Assessments include a thorough history and a physical examination; these are essential in identifying patients at risk or those with PAD.

Diagnosis is confirmed by non-invasive testing. Initially, bilateral arm and ankle systolic blood pressure is measured; as ankle pulses may be difficult to palpate, a Doppler probe may be placed over the dorsalis pedis or posterior tibial arteries. Ankle–brachial pressure index (ABPI) assessment assesses the patient's vascular status and determines if there is a presence of PAD by comparing systolic blood pressure at the ankle with the arm. A cuff is placed around each arm and ankle consecutively. ABPI testing can also be referred to as Doppler testing. The Doppler ultrasound is the traditional way of conducting an ABPI assessment. A Doppler uses high-frequency waves to measure the amount of blood flowing through the patient's veins and arteries. ABPI assessment can be used as a more accurate identification of people at potential risk of arterial disease including amputation, heart attack and stroke. Table 8.2 shows the interpretation of ABPI results.

The use of angiography provides details of the location and extent of arterial stenoses or occlusion. This must be performed prior to surgical correction or percutaneous transluminal angioplasty. Magnetic resonance angiography and computed tomography angiography are non-invasive alternatives to catheter contrast angiography.

The Fontaine classification is a system that is used to categorise the severity of PAD based on clinical symptoms and the ABPI. Using the Fontaine classification system can help clinicians to assess the severity of PAD and determine appropriate treatment strategies. The system considers both the patient's symptoms and the objective ABPI measurements. When

Table 8.2 Interpretation of ankle–brachial pressure index results (NICE 2023)

Less than 0.5	Suggests severe arterial disease.
Greater than 0.5 to less than 0.8	Suggests the presence of arterial disease or mixed arterial/venous disease.
Between 0.8 and 1.3	Suggests no evidence of significant arterial disease.
Greater than 1.3	This may suggest the presence of arterial calcification, such as in some people with diabetes, rheumatoid arthritis, systemic vasculitis, atherosclerotic disease and advanced chronic renal failure.

Table 8.3 Stages of peripheral arterial disease

Stage	Explanation
Stage I	Asymptomatic
	The patient has no symptoms or complaints related to peripheral arterial disease.
	Ankle–brachial pressure index (ABPI) is usually normal (greater than 0.9).
Stage II	Intermittent claudication
	The patient experiences intermittent claudication during physical activity, such as walking.
	ABPI may be reduced during exercise but typically normal at rest (between 0.7 and 0.9).
Stage III	Rest pain/nocturnal pain
	Moderate claudication. The patient experiences more severe claudication, limiting daily activities.
	ABPI is significantly reduced, often below 0.5, indicating reduced blood flow to the affected limb.

Stage	Explanation
Stage IV	Necrosis/gangrene
	Chronic limb-threatening ischaemia. This is the most severe stage, and patients may present with one or more of the following:
	• Rest pain: Persistent pain in the affected limb, especially when lying down.
	• Ulcers: Non-healing wounds or ulcers on the toes, feet or legs.
	• Gangrene: Tissue death may be present, which is a medical emergency.
	ABPI is usually severely reduced, often below 0.4.

Source: Adapted from Bunce, Ray, and Patel (2023); Aitken (2020).

assessed, treatment options can be determined; these range from lifestyle modifications and medications in the earlier stages (I and II) to more invasive interventions, for example, angioplasty, stenting or surgery in the later stages (III and IV). See Table 8.3 for a discussion of the various stages of PAD. Early detection and management are key in preventing complications and to improve the patients' quality of life.

MANAGEMENT

The treatment of PAD is guided by the disease severity (Tables 8.2 and 8.3). Aitkin (2020) notes that traditionally, treatment has focused on patients with symptoms of PAD. With increasing understanding, however, of the long-term morbidity and mortality consequences of PAD, a renewed emphasis on the importance of preventive therapy for asymptomatic patients is required.

All patients require intensive risk factor modification for relief of PAD symptoms and prevention of cardiovascular disease and avoidance of potential complications (see Box 8.2).

BOX 8.2 SOME COMPLICATIONS ASSOCIATED WITH PAD

PAD can lead to complications, which can include the following:

- Difficulty managing daily activities without help as a result of reduced mobility.
- Chronic inadequate blood flow to limbs (chronic limb-threatening ischaemia). Symptoms may include:
  - Pain during rest
  - Ulceration
  - Infection
  - Gangrene

(Continued)

BOX 8.2 (CONTINUED)

Gangrene is a severe complication that may require amputation of the affected body part.

- Serious infections: These may develop as a result of ulcers on the feet that then become infected. Infections in the foot can usually be treated with antibiotics; however, this may require treatment in a hospital if the infection is serious. The infection can also affect tissues and muscles, the bone and bloodstream. Bloodstream infections need to be treated immediately. The risk of these complications is higher for those with PAD and diabetes.
- When a sudden drop in blood flow to the limb occurs, this is known as acute limb ischaemia (see Table 8.1) and is a serious medical emergency. The person may suddenly lose feeling in the foot, they are unable to move it, it becomes blue or paler and colder than the other foot. Accessing treatment quickly may save the limb.
- Impairment of quality of life by claudication along with a reduction in mobility.
- Advanced PAD can result in psychosocial consequences such as depression.
- People with PAD are also at high risk of vascular complications, such as, myocardial infarction, stroke, vascular dementia, renal-related vascular disease and mesenteric disease.
- Atherosclerosis is often generalised, and if present at one site, there is an overall risk of cardiovascular events.

Source: Adapted from NICE (2020), Cea-Soriano et al. (2018) and Aboyans et al. (2018).

PHARMACOLOGICAL INTERVENTIONS

There are a range of prescribed medicines that are used to treat PAD and to prevent complications. These may include:

Antiplatelet medicines, for example, aspirin or clopidogrel, prevent blood clots from forming and narrowing the arteries even further. These medicines can also lower the risk of myocardial infarction or stroke. There are potential side effects associated with this group of medications; they include bleeding or an allergic reaction. An anticoagulant medicine (or blood thinner) such as rivaroxaban may be prescribed to help prevent blood clot formation.

Statins lower cholesterol and certain fats in the blood and can slow the progression of plaque build-up in the arteries that causes symptoms. Statins will also lower the risk of complications from PAD. Side effects are rare but may include muscle pain, indigestion, headaches and nausea.

ACE inhibitors and angiotensin II receptor blockers (ARBs) or other medicines lower blood pressure and prevent blood vessels from narrowing. ACE inhibitors block the actions of some hormones that help regulate blood pressure, which will decrease blood pressure. Side effects associated with ACE inhibitors include:

- Dizziness
- Tiredness or weakness
- Headaches
- A persistent dry cough

Most of these side effects will pass in a few days, although some people find they have a dry cough for longer. If the side effects become severe, a similar medicine called an ARB may be recommended.

Naftidrofuryl oxalate may be offered if the patient has leg pain that is triggered by exercise (intermittent claudication). This medicine may improve blood flow in the body and is very occasionally used if the patient prefers not to have surgery. It may also be used if the supervised exercise programme has not led to a satisfactory improvement in the person's condition. Side effects of naftidrofuryl oxalate may include:

- Nausea
- Abdominal pain
- Diarrhoea
- Rashes

Normally, patients are advised to take naftidrofuryl oxalate for around 3–6 months, to determine if its use improves symptoms. If the treatment is not effective after this time, it is stopped.

SURGICAL AND RADIOLOGICAL INTERVENTIONS

Vascular interventions for stable claudication are not generally advocated, except when the symptoms are severe or disabling (Bunce, Ray, and Patel 2023). A procedure to restore the flow of blood through the arteries in the legs may be recommended, which is known as revascularisation.

Revascularisation may be recommended if leg pain is so severe it prevents the person from undertaking everyday activities, or if symptoms have failed to respond to the treatments mentioned. There are two main types of revascularisation treatment for PAD:

- Percutaneous transluminal angioplasty – where a blocked or narrowed section of artery is widened by inflating a tiny balloon inside the vessel. Consideration may be given to the insertion of a stent; this is based on clinical need.
- Artery bypass graft – where blood vessels are taken from another part of the body and used to bypass the blockage in an artery.

There are advantages and disadvantages concerning either of the revascularisation approaches:

Percutaneous transluminal angioplasty is less invasive than a bypass. It does not involve large incisions and is usually performed under local anaesthetic as a procedure. Angioplasty is generally preferred to bypass surgery, unless angioplasty is not suitable or has previously failed. The results of a bypass, however, are generally thought to be longer-lasting than those of an angioplasty. This may mean that the procedure may need to be repeated less often than an angioplasty.

Both angioplasty and bypass surgery bring with them a small risk of serious complications, for example, myocardial infarction, stroke and even death. Before recommending a treatment option, options will be discussed with the patient; this will include the potential risks and benefits.

AMPUTATION

In severe ischaemia where there is unreconstructable arterial disease, an amputation may be necessary (Bunce, Ray, and Patel 2023). An amputation commonly leads to loss of independence and a significant impact on person's mental well-being. Amputation is a procedure of last resort and is indicated for uncontrolled infection, unrelenting rest pain and progressive gangrene (Menzies-Gow 2019). Amputation should be as distal as possible, preserving the knee for optimal use with a prosthesis.

MINOR AMPUTATION

In case of chronic limb-threatening ischaemia, minor amputation (up to the forefoot level) is often necessary to remove necrotic tissues with minor consequences on the patient's mobility. Revascularisation is needed prior to amputation to improve wound healing.

MAJOR AMPUTATION

Patients with extensive necrosis or infectious gangrene and those who are non-ambulatory with severe comorbidities may be best served with primary major amputation. Major amputation remains the last option to avoid or cease general complications of irreversible limb ischaemia; in some cases, this may allow patient recovery with rehabilitation and the use of prosthesis.

Secondary amputation should be performed when revascularisation has failed and re-intervention is no longer possible or when the limb continues to deteriorate because of infection or necrosis despite patent graft and optimal management.

PROGNOSIS

The course of PAD is not always predictable. It can progress gradually along a spectrum from claudication to rest pain to ischaemic ulcers or gangrene, but progression may be more sudden. Amputation is eventually required in around 1–2% of people with intermittent claudication. This increases to 5% in people with diabetes. Chronic limb-threatening ischaemia carries a high risk of amputation and premature death (Morley et al. 2018). Most people with PAD also have atherosclerotic disease of the brain or heart. They are three times more likely to die of cardiovascular causes than someone without PAD. Cardiovascular events are more likely in people with PAD, even if it is asymptomatic (NICE 2020).

HEALTH TEACHING

The two most important lifestyle changes that should be instigated as soon as a diagnosis is made are to exercise more regularly and if the person smokes, to stop smoking.

EXERCISE

Evidence suggests that regular exercise helps to reduce the severity and frequency of PAD symptoms, while also reducing the risk of developing another cardiovascular disease. Exercise can also boost self-esteem, mood, sleep quality and energy. NICE (2020) recommends supervised exercise as one of the first steps for managing PAD. This can involve group exercise sessions with other people with cardiovascular disease, these sessions are led by a trainer. Usually, the exercise programme involves two hours of supervised exercise a week for three months. The aim for the person to exercise daily, as the benefits of exercise are quickly lost if it is not frequent and regular.

Walking is one of the best exercises that can be done. It is usually recommended that the person walks as far and as long as they can before the symptoms of pain become intolerable. Then they should rest until the pain goes. Begin walking again until the pain returns. Use this 'stop-start' method until at least 30 minutes of walking in total has been achieved. This should be undertaken several times a week. The exercise course should improve symptoms.

STOP SMOKING

Stopping smoking will reduce the risk of PAD getting worse and another serious cardiovascular diseases from developing. Those who smoke after receiving their diagnosis are much more likely to have a heart attack and die from a complication of heart disease than people who quit after their diagnosis.

Smoking cessation provides the most noticeable improvement in walking distance when combined with regular exercise, particularly when lesions are located below the femoral arteries. In patients with intermittent claudication, ongoing tobacco use worsens the natural history of the condition, increasing the risk of amputation.

HEALTHY WEIGHT

Aim for a healthy weight. If overweight, losing just 3–5% of current weight can help manage some PAD risk factors, for example, hypertension, high blood cholesterol and diabetes. Losing even more weight can lower blood pressure further.

OTHER LIFESTYLE CHANGES

In addition to exercising and stopping smoking, a number of other lifestyle changes can be made to reduce the risk of developing other forms of cardiovascular disease. These include the following:

- Eating a balanced diet.
- Managing weight.
- Cutting down on alcohol consumption.

MENTAL WELL-BEING

PAD can cause severe pain and disrupt a person's life. If the person is experiencing depression or anxiety access to support should be arranged. Learning how to manage stress, relax, get good-quality sleep and cope with problems can improve emotional and physical health.

DIABETES

Having poorly controlled diabetes can also make the symptoms of PAD worse and increase the risk of developing other forms of cardiovascular disease. It is important that people with diabetes are managed effectively, which may involve lifestyle changes. These could include eating a healthy, balanced diet and taking medicines to lower blood glucose levels.

Foot care is important for people with PVD, for example, daily foot inspection, keeping ischaemic feet clean to avoid infection, being careful to avoid injury when cutting the toenails, avoiding walking barefoot and wearing well-fitting shoes. Referral to a chiropodist may be needed.

The patient should be directed to the Driver and Vehicle Licencing Agency for more information regarding driving. See the Driver and Vehicle Licensing Agency (2023) publication 'Assessing Fitness to Drive: A Guide for Medical Professionals'.

CONCLUSION

PAD is a major contributor to the mortality and morbidity of patients with atherosclerosis in the UK. For those with chronic limb-threatening ischaemia, revascularisation is the basis of limb salvage as well as accelerated access to vascular surgery assessment is essential.

GLOSSARY OF TERMS

Angiography: An invasive procedure that uses contrast dye and X-rays to visualise the blood vessels, often performed for precise assessment of arterial blockages.

Angioplasty: An interventional procedure involving the inflation of a balloon-like device within a narrowed artery to widen it and improve blood flow.

Ankle–brachial pressure index: A non-invasive test that measures blood pressure in the ankle and arm to assess the severity of arterial blockages in the lower extremities.

Antiplatelet agents: Medications, such as aspirin and clopidogrel, inhibit platelet aggregation and help prevent blood clots.

Atherosclerosis: The build-up of plaque (fatty deposits, cholesterol and other substances) within the arteries, leading to reduced blood flow.

Bypass surgery: A surgical procedure that reroutes blood flow around blocked or narrowed arteries to improve blood supply to the extremities.

Chronic limb-threatening ischaemia: Previously known as critical limb ischaemia. The most severe stage of peripheral arterial disease, characterised by rest pain, ulcers or gangrene due to severely restricted blood flow.

Cyanosis: Bluish discolouration of the skin, often indicating poor oxygenation of tissues.

Doppler ultrasound: A diagnostic test that uses sound waves to evaluate blood flow within blood vessels, including those affected by peripheral arterial disease.

Fontaine classification: A staging system used to categorise the severity of peripheral arterial disease based on clinical symptoms and ABPI measurements.

Gangrene: The death of tissue due to a lack of blood supply, which can be a severe complication of peripheral arterial disease.

Intermittent claudication: Muscle pain, cramping or discomfort in the legs during physical activity, such as walking, due to reduced blood flow.

Ischaemia: Inadequate blood supply to tissues, leading to oxygen and nutrient deprivation, which can cause damage or cell death.

Lifestyle modifications: Behavioural changes such as smoking cessation, dietary changes, exercise and weight management aimed at improving overall health and managing peripheral arterial disease.

Pallor: Paleness of the skin due to reduced blood flow or oxygenation.

Peripheral arterial disease: A circulatory disorder characterised by the narrowing or blockage of arteries that supply blood to the extremities, primarily the legs.

Risk factors: Factors that increase the likelihood of developing peripheral arterial disease, including smoking, diabetes, hypertension and family history.

Revascularisation: Medical procedures or surgeries aimed at restoring blood flow to areas affected by peripheral arterial disease.

Statins: Medications prescribed to lower cholesterol levels and reduce the risk of atherosclerosis progression.

Stenting: The placement of a small mesh tube (stent) in a narrowed artery to keep it open and maintain blood flow.

Ulcers: Non-healing wounds or open sores on the extremities, often observed in severe cases of peripheral arterial disease.

MULTIPLE CHOICE QUESTIONS

1. What is the primary cause of peripheral arterial disease (PAD)?
   a) Hypertension
   b) Atherosclerosis
   c) Diabetes
   d) Smoking

2. Which symptom is characteristic of PAD early stages?
   a) Rest pain
   b) Muscle atrophy
   c) Intermittent claudication
   d) Gangrene

3. Which diagnostic test measures blood pressure in the ankle and arm to assess PAD severity?
   a) Echocardiogram
   b) Electrocardiogram (ECG)
   c) Ankle–brachial pressure index (ABPI)
   d) Magnetic resonance imaging

4. Which Fontaine classification stage represents asymptomatic PAD?
   a) Stage I
   b) Stage II
   c) Stage III
   d) Stage IV

5. What lifestyle modification is important for PAD management?
   a) Smoking cessation
   b) Increasing saturated fat intake
   c) Sedentary lifestyle
   d) Excessive alcohol consumption

6. Which medication is often prescribed to reduce cholesterol levels in PAD patients?
   a) Antibiotics
   b) Diuretics
   c) Statins
   d) Anticoagulants

7. In PAD, which skin change may be observed due to reduced blood flow?
   a) Erythema (redness)
   b) Pallor (paleness)
   c) Petechiae
   d) Excessive sweating

8. What does ABPI stand for in the context of PAD diagnosis?
   a) Ankle blood pressure index
   b) Arterial blockage pressure indicator
   c) Ankle–brachial pressure index
   d) Aortic blood pressure index

9. Which medication is commonly used to prevent blood clots in PAD patients?
   a) Aspirin
   b) Ibuprofen
   c) Acetaminophen
   d) Antibiotics

10. In PAD, what is the term for non-healing wounds or open sores on the extremities?
    a) Ulcers
    b) Plaques
    c) Aneurysms
    d) Embolisms

REFERENCES

Aboyans, V., Ricco, J.B., Bartelink, M.E.L. et al. (2018). 2017 ESC guidelines on the diagnosis and treatment of peripheral arterial diseases, in collaboration with the European Society for Vascular Surgery (ESVS): document covering atherosclerotic disease of extracranial carotid and vertebral, mesenteric, renal, upper and lower extremity arteries. Endorsed by: The European Stroke Organization (ESO). The task force for the diagnosis and treatment of peripheral arterial diseases of the European Society of Cardiology (ESC) and of the European Society for Vascular Surgery (ESVS). *European Heart Journal* 39 (9): 763–816.

Aitken, S.J. (2020). Peripheral artery disease in the lower limbs: the importance of secondary risk prevention for improved long-term prognosis. *Australian Journal of General Practice* 49 (5): 239–244. doi:10.31128/AJGP-11-19-5160.

Bunce, N.H., Ray, R., and Patel, H. (2023). Cardiology (Chapter 30). In: *Kumar and Clark's Clinical Medicine,* 10e (eds. A. Feather, D. Randall, and M. Waterhouse). London: Elsevier.

Cea-Soriano, L., Fowkes, F.G.R., Johansson, S. et al. (2018). Time trends in peripheral artery disease incidence, prevalence and secondary preventive therapy: a cohort study in the Health Improvement Network in the UK. *BMJ Open* 8 (1): e018184. https://e018184.full.pdf (bmj.com).

Driver and Vehicle Licensing Agency. (2023). *Assessing Fitness to Drive: A Guide for Medical Professionals.* https://www.gov.uk/government/publications/ assessing-fitness-to-drive-a-guide-for-medicalprofessionals (accessed October 2023).

Farber, A. (2018). Chronic limb-threatening ischemia. *New England Journal of Medicine* 379 (2): 171–180.

Gerhard-Herman, M.D., Gornik, H.L., Barrett, C. et al. (2017). 2016 AHA/ACC guideline on the management of patients with lower extremity peripheral artery disease: a report of the American College of Cardiology/American Heart Association Task Force on Clinical Practice Guidelines. *Circulation* 135 (12): e726–e779. doi: 10.1161/CIR.0000000000000471.

Hagler, D., Harding, M.M., Kwang, J. et al. (2023). *Lewis's Medical-Surgical Nursing*, 12e. St Louis: Elsevier.

Menzies-Gow, E. (2019). Nursing patients with cardiovascular disorders (Chapter 3). In: *Alexander's Nursing Practice,* 5e (ed. I. Peate). London: Elsevier.

Mills, N.L., Japp, A.G., and Robson, J. (2018). The cardiovascular system (Chapter 4). In: *MacLeod's Clinical Examination,* 14e (eds. J.A. Innes, A.R. Dover, and K. Fairhurst). London: Elsevier.

Mitchell, A. (2023). Peripheral arterial disease (Chapter 44). In: *Long Term Conditions in Adults at a Glance.* (eds. A. Mitchell, B. Hill, and I. Peate). Oxford: Wiley.

Morley, R.L., Sharma, A., Horsch, A.D. et al. (2018). Peripheral artery disease. *British Medical Journal* 360: j5842.

National Institute for Health and Care Excellence. (2020). *Peripheral Arterial Disease: Diagnosis and Management.* Peripheral arterial disease: diagnosis and management. https://www.nice.org.uk/Guidance/CG147 (accessed October 2023).

National Institute for Health and Care Excellence. (2023). *How Should I Interpret Ankle Brachial Pressure Index (ABPI) Results*? Interpretation of ABPI | Diagnosis | Leg ulcer - venous | CKS | NICE. (accessed October 2021).

Rajan, R., Jayakumar, R.B., Al-Jarallah, M. et al. (2022). Diabetes and peripheral artery disease. *e-Journal of Cardiology Practice,* 22: 13. https://www.escardio.org/Journals/E-Journal-of-Cardiology-Practice/Volume-22/diabetes-and-peripheral-artery-disease.

MCQ Answers

Chapter 1   Anatomy and Physiology: The Cardiovascular System
1. (c); 2. (c); 3. (a); 4. (b); 5. (b); 6. (b); 7. (a); 8. (b); 9. (a); 10. (c).

Chapter 2   Cardiovascular Assessment
1. (b); 2. (b); 3. (c); 4. (b); 5. (c); 6. (c); 7. (c); 8. (b); 9. (b); 10. (b).

Chapter 3   Myocardial Infarction
1. (b); 2. (c); 3. (a); 4. (d); 5. (a); 6. (a); 7. (d); 8. (c); 9. (c); 10. (c).

Chapter 4   Heart Failure
1. (c); 2. (d); 3. (c); 4. (c); 5. (c); 6. (c); 7. (c); 8. (c); 9. (a); 10. (b).

Chapter 5   Cardiogenic Shock
1. (c); 2. (c); 3. (b); 4. (c); 5. (d); 6. (a); 7. (b); 8. (b); 9. (a); 10. (b).

Chapter 6   Angina
1. (c); 2. (a); 3. (c); 4. (a); 5. (b); 6. (c); 7. (b); 8. (c); 9. (b); 10. (d).

Chapter 7   Hypertension
1. (c); 2. (a); 3. (a); 4. (c); 5. (a); 6. (d); 7. (b); 8. (c); 9. (b); 10. (c).

Chapter 8   Peripheral Arterial Disease
1. (b); 2. (c); 3. (c); 4. (a); 5. (a); 6. (c); 7. (b); 8. (c); 9. (a); 10. (a).

Index

Note: Page numbers in *italics* and **bold** refers to figures and tables respectively.

A

ABO blood groups, 6
acute coronary syndrome, 39, 53
acute kidney injury (AKI), 85
acute limb ischaemia, **129**
acute myocardial infarction, 46, 53, 86
acute respiratory distress syndrome (ARDS), 85
adenosine triphosphate (ATP), 85
adrenaline, 114
adult(s)
   with acute coronary syndrome, 53
   basic life support guidelines, 81–83
   sequence of basic adult life support, *84*
afterload, 64, 87
age/ageing
   heart failure changes with, 68
   with hypertension, 116, **116**
   as risk factor of angina, 101
air pollution, as risk factor of angina, 101
albumin, 4
alcohol consumption associated with hypertension, **116**, 117–118
aldosterone, 114
amputation, 135
   major, 136
   minor, 136
aneurysm, 118
angina, 51, 96
   age, 101
   clinical investigations and diagnosis, 103
   clinical presentation, 103
   due to air pollution, 101
   epidemiology, 101
   ethnicity, 102
   family history, 101
   gender, 102
   genetics, 101
   health teaching, 107–108
   lifestyle habits, 102
   management, 104
   medical procedures, 102
   microvascular angina, 98–99
   other interventions, 107
   other medical conditions, 102
   pathophysiological changes associated with, 99–101
   pharmacological interventions, 105–106, **105**, *107*
   PQRST assessment of, **103**
   Prinzmetal's angina, 98
   risk factors, 101
   silent, 97–98
   stable, 96–97
   tests and investigations, **104**
angina pectoris. *see* angina
angiography, 132
angioplasty, 135
angiotensin-converting enzyme inhibitors (ACE inhibitors), 54, 72, 104, 123
   reduce cardiovascular risk, 128
   side effects associated with, 134
angiotensin II receptor blockers (ARBs), 123, 134
ankle–brachial pressure index (ABPI), 131
   interpretation of, **132**
anorexia, 70
anticoagulant medicine, 134
anti-hypertensive medicines
   angiotensin-converting enzyme inhibitors, 123
   angiotensin II receptor blockers, 123
   beta-blockers, 124
   calcium channel blockers, 123
   diuretics, 123
antiplatelet
   drugs for angina, 104
   drugs for myocardial infarction, 53
   medicines, 134
   therapy for symptomatic PAD, 128
   treatments, 54
anxiety, 118
aorta, 13
aortic aneurysms, 118
arrhythmia, 48, 53, 64
arrhythmogenic right ventricular dysplasia, 81
arterial blood gas analysis, 89
arterial hypertension, 116
arteries, 6, 7–8
   comparison of vein, capillary and, 9
   structure and function of, 7
artery bypass graft, 135
aspirin, 134
atheromatous plaque, 46
atherosclerosis, *46*, 109, 120, 130, 134
atherosclerotic arterial narrowing, 101
atherosclerotic plaques in coronary arteries, 96
atrial fibrillation, 3, 42, 66–67, *66*
atrioventricular (AV) node, 17
atrioventricular (AV) valves, 12
automated electronic defibrillator (AED), 82–83
autonomic nervous system, 114
AV bundle. *see* Bundle of His

B

baroreceptor(s), 114
   reflex, 114
beta-blockers
   angina, 104, **105**
   anti-hypertensive medicines, 123
   heart failure and, 65, 72
   myocardial infarction and, 53, 54
bicuspid (mitral) valve, 12
blood, 1–6
   appearance of centrifuged, 3

143

144 Index

clot, 47
components of, 5
composition of, 1–4
flow through heart, 14–15
formed elements of, 3
general functions, 1
groups, 5–6
properties of, 4
tests, 72
blood cells
formation of, 4
types, **2**
blood pressure (BP), 113–114
correct positioning of cuff, *120*
equation, 115
guide to cardiovascular risk, 33–34
measurement in diagnosing hypertension, 120–121
readings, **114**
sphygmomanometer and stethoscope, *120*
blood vessels, 1, 6–10
of heart, 13, 15
layers of, 8
vessel resistance, 114
bradycardia, 33, 89
British Heart Foundation (BHF), 48
Brugada syndrome, 81
B-type natriuretic peptide (BNP), 72
bundle branches, cardiac conduction system, 18
Bundle of His, cardiac conduction system, 18
bypass surgery, 135

C

calcium channel blockers
as anti-hypertensive medicines, 123
exacerbate pre-existing heart failure, 65
pharmacological approaches to angina, 104, **105**
capillaries, 6, 9
comparison of vein, artery and, 9
capillary filling time, 86
capillary nail refill test, 29
capillary refill time, 29–30
measurement of capillary nail bed refill, 30
cardiac arrest, 79
epidemiology, 80, **80**

guidelines for adult basic life support, 81–83
risk factors associated with, 81
cardiac auscultation, 35–36
points, *36*
cardiac catheterisation, 72, 107
cardiac chest pain, 39
cardiac conduction, 17
cardiac cycle, 18–19, 115, *115*
cardiac output
arterial hypertension in, 116
cardiogenic shock results in low, 86
pathophysiological changes associated with heart failure, 62
cardiac pain, 39
areas associated with, *41*
inferences made regarding, **41**
cardiac radionuclide scan, 71
cardiac rehabilitation, 56, 107
cardiac shock. *see* cardiogenic shock
cardiac syndrome X. *see* microvascular angina
cardiogenic shock, 58, 79, **84**, *91*
clinical investigations and diagnosis, 89
clinical presentation, 89
epidemiology, 87
management, 90, **90**
mechanisms associated with, **87**
pathophysiological changes associated with, 86–87
physiotherapist, 92
potential investigations, 89
risk factors, 88, **88**
cardiomegaly, 75
cardiomyopathies, 64
cardiovascular assessment, 24
assessing chest pain, 39–41
blood pressure, 33–34
chest examination, 34–36
chief complaint and history of present condition, 27
common manifestations of cardiovascular problems, **29**
electrocardiogram, 36–38
family history, 27
importance of, 24
indicated, **24–25**
lifestyle, 28
needs, 25–26
palpation, 29–33

past medical history, 28
physical examination, 28–29
cardiovascular changes, 85
cardiovascular disease, 49
comorbidities increase risk of, 51
modifiable and non-modifiable risk factors for developing, **50**
and PAD, 130, 136
social deprivation, 50
South Asian and Black groups at higher risk of, 50
in UK, 67
cardiovascular system
blood, 1–6
heart, 10–19
catecholamines, 87
cellular hypoxia, 85
cerebral oedema, 79
chamber dilation, **63**
chest examination, 34–36
chest pain. *see also* angina
assessment, 39–41
OLDCARTS chest pain assessment, **40**
possible causes of, **40**
chest X-ray
cardiogenic shock, 89
investigation of heart failure, 53, 72
cholesterol-lowering agents, 54
chronic heart failure, 68
chronic kidney disease, 119, 130
chronic limb-threatening ischaemia, 128, **129**, 130, 131, 133, 136
chronic stable angina, 96
chronic stress
on heart, **63**
impact heart health, 91
circulation, blood, 1
circulatory system. *see* cardiovascular system
Civil Aviation Authority
Assessing fitness to fly: Guidelines for health professionals, 74
claudication, 130
vascular interventions for stable, 135
clinical assessment skills, 24
clopidogrel, 134
coagulation, 85
collagen, 47

commence cardiopulmonary resuscitation (CPR), 81–82
compensatory mechanisms, 86–87
computed tomography angiography, 132
conducting system, 17–18
congenital heart disease, 64
congestive cardiac failure, 62
congestive heart failure, 62
   signs of, 53
coronary angiography, 89
coronary angioplasty. *see* percutaneous coronary intervention (PCI)
coronary arteries, 16
   atherosclerotic plaques in, 96
coronary artery bypass, 104
coronary artery bypass grafting (CABG), 102, 107
coronary artery disease
   angina caused by, 96
   blockage of, *97*
coronary circulation, 15
coronary heart disease (CHD), 46
coronary sinus, 16–17
coronary thrombosis, 46
coronary veins, 16
critical limb ischaemia. *see* chronic limb-threatening ischaemia
CT coronary angiography, 53
cyanosis, 28–29, 70, 138

D
delayed capillary refill time, 30
deprivation, hypertension impact of, 118
diabetes
   HbA1C test for, 122
   heart attacks and, 49
   increased risk of PAD, 130, 137–138
   increased risk of silent angina, 98
   modifiable and non-modifiable risk factors for, **50**
   risk factors associated with cardiogenic shock, **88**
   risk factors for cardiovascular disease, 50, 51
   in South Asian and Black groups, 50
diabetes mellitus. *see* diabetes
diastole
   first phase, 18
   second phase, 19
diastolic blood pressure, 113, 114

distended jugular veins, 69
distributive shock, **84**, 86
diuretics, 72, 123
Doppler ultrasound, 132
Driver and Vehicle Licensing Agency, 74
dyspnoea, 42
   chest pain and, 51
   paroxysmal nocturnal, 27
   signs and symptoms of right-sided heart failure, 70

E
echocardiography
   cardiogenic shock, 89
   clinical investigations for MI, 53
   tests and investigations for heart failure, 71
ejection fraction
   heart failure with preserved, 62
   heart failure with reduced, 62
electrocardiogram (ECG), 36–38
   for cardiogenic shock, 90
   changes during episode of Prinzmetal's angina, 98
   chest lead placement, *37*
   for ischaemia, 97
   for MI, 46–47
   performing, 39
   placement of limb leads, *38*
   12-lead normal, *38*
elevated blood pressure, 116
embolus, 58
endocardium, 12
end of life care, 73
endothelial dysfunction, 85
erythrocytes. *see* red blood cells
essential hypertension. *see* primary hypertension
ethnicity
   for angina, 102
   with hypertension, **116**, 117
   myocardial infarction and, 50
   risk of heart failure, 67
European Society of Cardiology, 62
excess dietary salt with hypertension, 117
exercise
   aerobic, 118
   cardiac rehabilitation and, 107
   claudication and, 128
   for PAD symptoms, 136–137
   silent angina during, 97
   stress test, 103

   taking as self-management programmes, 107–108
   tolerance test, 72
extracellular matrix alterations, **63**
eye damage, hypertension and, 119

F
family history
   cardiovascular assessment, 27
   of kidney failure, 119
   as risk factor of angina, 101
fibrinogen, 4
fibrous pericardium, 10
fluid shifts, 85
Fontaine classification system, 132
foot care for PVD patient, 137
foreign body airway obstruction, 83

G
gangrene, 128, 131, 134
gender
   and angina, 102
   with hypertension, **116**, 117
general practitioner (GP), 27, 67, 123
genetics
   as risk factor of angina, 101
   role in hypertension, 117
globulins, 4
glyceryl trinitrate (GTN), 98, 106
graft surgery, 104

H
haemodynamic changes, **63**
haemodynamic equation, 115
haemopoiesis, 5
haemoptysis, 70
HbA1C test, 121
Health Survey for England, 116
   modifiable and non-modifiable risk factors with hypertension, **116**
health teaching
   for angina, 107–108
   heart failure, 73–74
   in hypertension, 124
   myocardial infarction, 55
   in peripheral arterial disease, 136–138
healthy lifestyle adaptation for control hypertension, 123
healthy weight
   physically active aiming for, 107
   reducing PAD risk factors, 137
   reducing strain on heart, 91

Index

heart, 1, 10
   blood flow through, 14–15
   blood vessels of, 13, 15
   chambers of, 12, 13
   conducting system of, 17
   location of, 11
   valves of, 12
   walls of, 10, 11
heart attack. *see* myocardial infarction (MI)
heart failure, 48, 49, 62
   atrial fibrillation, 66–67
   causes of, 64–65
   classification of severity of, **69**
   clinical investigations and diagnosis, 70
   clinical presentation, 68–69
   complications associated with, **66**
   congestive, 53
   end of life care, 73
   epidemiology, 67
   health teaching, 73–74
   heart failure changes with ageing, 68
   hypertension and, 119
   left-sided heart failure, signs and symptoms of, 70
   management, 72–73
   pathophysiological changes associated with, 62, **63**
   red flags for, *70*
   right-sided heart failure, signs and symptoms of, 69–70
   risk factors, 67–68, **68**
   signs and symptoms associated with, *71*
heart failure with preserved ejection fraction (HFpEF), 62
   women commonly causes by, 67
heart failure with reduced ejection fraction (HFrEF), 62
   men causes by, 67
heart-healthy diet, 91
heart-healthy eating pattern, 107
heart rate, irregular, 27
hepatic dysfunction, 85
hepatomegaly, 69
history taking
   systematic approach to, 25–26
   usual sequence of events, *26*
hypercholesterolaemia, 130
hypertension, 113
   blood pressure, 113–114
   blood pressure measurement, 120–121

cardiac cycle, 115, *115*
clinical investigations and diagnosis, 121–122
clinical presentation, 118–121
complications of, *119*
depending on extent of MI, 52
epidemiology, 116
family history of, 27
health teaching, 124
heart failure, 64
management, 122–124
pathophysiological changes associated with, 116
and peripheral arterial disease, 130
primary and secondary, 113
risk factors, 116
white coat syndrome, 121
hypertrophy, **63**
hypoperfusion, 85
hypotension. *see also* hypertension
   in cardiovascular assessment, 27
   depending on extent of MI, 52
   in myocardial infarction, 48
   postural, 121
   shock leads to, 85
   venous vasodilator causing, 54
hypovolaemic shock, **84**
hypoxaemia, 93

I

identical twins, blood groups, 5–6
illicit drug use
   history of, 48–49
   leading to cardiac arrest, 81
increased afterload conditions, **63**
infarct, 47
in-hospital cardiac arrest (IHCA), **80**
intermittent claudication, 128, 131
intravenous (IV) infusion, 54
invasive strategy, 54
ischaemia, 46–47, 97
   acute limb ischaemia, **129**
   chronic limb-threatening ischaemia, **129**, 130, 131, 133
   limb, **129**
ischaemic heart disease, 40, 101

L

lactic acidosis, 85
left-sided heart failure, signs and symptoms of, 70
left ventricular failure, 62
leucocytes. *see* white blood cells
lifestyle

cardiovascular assessment and, 28
   risk factors for angina, 102
lifestyle changes, 124, 125
   angina, 107
   for cardiac events, 92
   for PAD, 136–137
   prevent and lower high BP, 124
   reducing risk of cardiovascular disease, 137
lifestyle modifications. *see* lifestyle changes
limb ischaemia, **129**
long QT syndrome, 81

M

magnetic resonance angiography, 132
major amputation, 136
medical history, 121
medical procedures, for angina, 102
men
   angina affects, 102
   blood volume of, 4
   heart attack rate in UK, 48
   heart failure in, 67
   heart size in, 10
mental health, hypertension and, 118
mental well-being, PAD and, 137
metered aerosol GTN spray, 106
microthrombi, 85
microvascular angina, 98–99
minor amputation, 136
modifiable risk factors with hypertension, **116**, 117–118
morphine, 54
MRI scan, for heart failure, 71
multidisciplinary team approach, 72
multiple organ dysfunction syndrome (MODS), 86
myocardial contractile dysfunction, **63**
myocardial disease, 64
myocardial dysfunction, 85
myocardial infarction (MI), 46, *48*, 62, 79, 99
   angina and, **99–100**
   areas of pain associated with, *52*
   atherosclerosis, *46*
   with cardiogenic shock, **88**
   clinical investigations, 53
   clinical presentation, 51–53

coronary artery disease
depicting healthy heart,
angina pectoris and, *100*
diagnosis, 53
epidemiology, 48
ethnicity, 50
family history of, 27
health teaching, 55
hypertension and, 119
lifestyle discussion points
following, **56–57**
management, 53
medication and, **54**
pathophysiological changes
associated with, 46–48
people with learning
disabilities, 49
presentation and clinical
features, 52
reperfusion, 54–55
risk factors, 50–51
ruptured atherosclerotic
plaque, *46*
social deprivation, 50
women, 49
younger patients, 48–49
myocardial ischaemia, 47
myocardial perfusion imaging. *see*
cardiac radionuclide scan
myocardium, 11–12, 46
cells of, 12

N
naftidrofuryl oxalate, 135
nail blanch test. *see* capillary nail
refill test
National Health Service, 67
National Institute for Health and
Care Excellence (NICE),
34, 53, 70, 96, 113
nausea condition in heart
failure, 70
neurohormonal activation, **63**
New York Heart Association
(NYHA), 65
nitrates, 104, **105**
chest pain treated with, 54
nitroglycerin [GTN], 99
non-modifiable risk factors with
hypertension, 116–117, **116**
non-steroidal anti-
inflammatory drugs, 65
non-ST-segment-elevation MI
(NSTEMI), 46
reperfusion, 53
normal coronary arteries, 98
N-terminal pro-B-type natriuretic
peptide (NT-proBNP), 72

nuclear cardiology scan. *see*
cardiac radionuclide scan

O
obesity
causes of heart failure, 65
with hypertension, **116**, 117
poor prognostic indicators, 65
risk factors associated with
cardiogenic shock, **88**
occupation, as risk factor of
angina, 101
oedema, 69
peripheral, 73
pulmonary, 72
OLDCARTS chest pain
assessment, 40, **40**
organ dysfunction and failure, 85
orthopnoea, 27, 70
out-of-hospital cardiac arrest
(OHCA), **80**

P
pallor, 131
palpation, 29
capillary refill time, 29–30
pulse, 30–33
paroxysmal nocturnal
dyspnoea, 27, 75
patient-centred approach, 56
people with learning disabilities,
myocardial infarction in, 49
percutaneous coronary
intervention (PCI), 48,
102, 107, *108*
percutaneous transluminal
angioplasty, 135
pericardial disease, 64
pericardium, 10
peripheral arterial disease
(PAD), 128
amputation, 135–136
clinical investigations and
diagnosis, 131
clinical presentation, 131
complications associated with
PAD, 133–134
epidemiology, 130
health teaching, 136–138
limb ischaemia, **129**
lower limb arteries, *129*
management, 133
pathophysiological changes
associated with PAD, 128
pharmacological
interventions, 134–135
prognosis, 136
risk factors, 130

stages of, **132–133**
surgical and radiological
interventions, 135
peripheral artery disease, 119
peripheral oedema, 27, 69, 73
peripheral vascular disease (PVD).
see peripheral arterial
disease (PAD)
peripheral vascular resistance
(PVR), 115
peripheral venous disease, 128
physical activity
essential for cardiovascular
health, 91
lack leads to hypertension, 118
physiotherapist
cardiac rehabilitation
conduct by, 56
cardiogenic shock and, 92
plasma, 4
platelets, 2
pleural effusion, 69
PQRST assessment of angina, **103**
preload, 75, **88**, 93
primary cardiac dysfunction, 79
primary hypertension, 113
Prinzmetal's angina, 98, 101
Public Health England (PHE), 48
pulmonary circulation, 14
pulmonary oedema, 53, 70,
71, 72, 87
pulse, 30–33
assessing radial, *32*
palpating dorsalis pedis, *32*
palpating popliteal pulse, *32*
palpating posterior tibial, *32*
peripheral, **31**, 34
Purkinje fibres, 18

R
ranolazine, 106
red blood cells, 2, 5
renin–angiotensin–aldosterone
system (RAAS), **63**
reperfusion, 54–55
coronary stent insertion, *55*
for NSTEMI, 53
for STEMI, 53
Resuscitation Council UK
(RCUK), 83
revascularisation, 135
rhythm of pulses, 33
right-sided heart failure, signs and
symptoms of, 69–70
right ventricular failure, 62
risk factors
of angina, 101–102
with cardiac arrest, 81

with cardiogenic shock, 88, **88**
for heart failure, 67–68, **68**
with hypertension, 116
modifiable risk factors, **116**, 117–118
for myocardial infarction, 50–51
non-modifiable risk factors, 116–117, **116**
with peripheral arterial disease, 130
rivaroxaban, 134

S
Scientific Advisory Committee on Nutrition (SACN), 117
Scottish Intercollegiate Guidelines Network (SIGN), 103
secondary amputation, 136
secondary hypertension, 113, 121
self-management programmes, 107–108
sepsis, 86
serial cardiac markers, 53
serial dynamic ECGs, 53
serous pericardium, 10
severe hypertension, 118
shock, 83. *see also* cardiogenic shock
signs and symptoms, 86
types of, **84**, 85–86
silent angina, 97–98
silent ischaemia angina. *see* silent angina
sinoatrial (SA) node, 16, 17
smoking
cessation and PAD, 137
quitting to improve heart health, 91
risk factors for PAD, 130
social deprivation, myocardial infarction and, 50
socioeconomic status, hypertension impact of, 118
South Asian and Black groups
diabetes prevalence and mortality in, 50
at higher risk of cardiovascular disease, 50
with highest mortality from heart disease, 102
sphygmomanometer, *120*
splenomegaly, 69
stable angina, 96–97
statins, 54, 104, 128, 134

stenting, 133
stent placement, 102, 107
stethoscope, *120*
for auscultation, 35
'stop-start' method, 137
stress, 118. *see also* hypertension
activation of stress response, 85
chronic, **63**, 91
echocardiography, 53
emotional, 96, 98
management techniques, 91, 137
risk factors for angina, 102
testing, 103, **104**
stroke
hypertension and, 118
mortality related to, 50
volume, 85, 125
structured assessment of chest pain, 39
ST-segment-elevation MI (STEMI), 46
reperfusion, 53
sudden cardiac arrest, 79
sympathetic nervous system, 114
sympathetic nervous system activation, **63**
symptomatic PAD, 130
systemic circulation, 15
systemic inflammation, 86
systemic inflammatory response syndrome (SIRS), 86
systole, 35
first phase, 19
second phase, 19
systolic blood pressure, 113, 114

T
tachycardia, 33, 70, 85
tachypnoea, 70
target organ damage, 121, 122
thrombocytes. *see* platelets
thrombus, 46, *47*
tissue perfusion, 85, 86
tricuspid valve, 12
troponin, 47, 93
tunica externa, 7
tunica interna, 7
tunica media, 7
12-lead electrocardiogram, 53, 72
type 2 diabetes, 117

U
ulcer/ulceration, 128
in PAD, 131, 133, 136
uncontrolled hypertension, 118

undiagnosed hypertension, 118
unstable angina, 96

V
valve disease, heart failure due to, 62
valvular disease, 96
valvular heart disease, 64
variant angina. *see* Prinzmetal's angina
vascular dementia, 119
vasoconstriction, 42
vasodilation, 42
vasodilators, 54
vasospasm, 98
vasospastic angina. *see* Prinzmetal's angina
veins, 6, 8–9
comparison of artery, capillary and, 9
network, 10
structure and function of, 7
venae cavae, 13
venous return, 42
ventricular remodelling, **63**
volume overload, **63**

W
walking, 136–137
white blood cells, 2
white coat effect. *see* white coat syndrome
white coat hypertension. *see* white coat syndrome
white coat syndrome, 121
women
angina affects, 102
blood volume of, 4
heart attack rate in UK, 48
heart failure in, 67
heart size in, 10
microvascular angina, 102
myocardial infarction in, 49

X
xanthelasma, 29

Y
younger patients
heart disease at, 102
myocardial infarction in, 48–49